FOOD
SOBRIETY

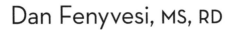

Dan Fenyvesi, MS, RD

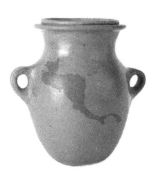

CONTENTS

FOREWORD

What If I Actually Do This?

by Jennifer Rodriguez Moran

The Facebook post read: "Hi friends. I'm looking for an illustrator to come work by my side in Nicaragua, to illustrate my book on weight loss and nutrition." I set down my cocktail and chips and re-read the message. My heart fluttered as I immediately typed "interested." And then I thought, what if I actually do this?

I got up and looked at myself in the mirror. I was 35 years old, and in the worst shape of my life. At 203 pounds I was obese, doctors told me. I wore stretchy pants and loose tops. I refused to buy myself anything new to wear until I needed a smaller size again. But I just kept growing. My size 16 clothes were getting too tight. My self-confidence was at an all-time low. Where did this body come from?

I lived in Chicago and walked or rode my bike to get around. I skipped the elevator and ran up and down the stairs. I got winded, but I did it. I was a dedicated foodie and amateur chef. I went to farmers' markets and food co-ops. I spent all of my money on the healthiest ingredients. Why was I so fat and unhappy?

Fast-forward six months. While we sat next to a shimmering pool in tropical Nicaragua, Dan asked me these same questions. Why was I feeling unhealthy? What exactly was I eating and doing? Then he began to explain to me the science behind weight loss and the lessons he learned from working in Nicaragua, which I sum up as "the path to health is far simpler and cheaper than we ever imagined." I listened eagerly to every

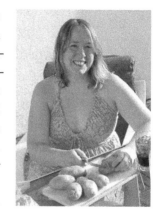

Before leaving for Nicaragua I weighed 203 pounds.

word he said. I was ready for a change. I was not willing to give up on my life! I wanted to climb mountains and trees, learn how to dance and surf, be strong enough to be a mom someday.

He passed me his manuscript. He instructed me to read, sketch, take notes. I found Dan's narrative to be funny at times, sad sometimes, true all the time.

I filled my notebook with illustration ideas. While we worked on the art, we were living the ideals Dan puts forth in Food Sobriety. We played soccer with the neighborhood kids. We cooked and ate together, using his simple recipes and fresh ingredients. We went surfing, hiking, and dancing with friends. Days and nights were filled with activity: illustrating, sketching, and debating ideas. We were making conscious decisions about how we were spending prime personal resources — our energy, time, and money. We were living life truly involved.

Then (for the first time since high school gym class), this 35-year-old put on the brand-new running shoes that until this trip had been languishing in my closet in Chicago. Dan and I often went jogging in the streets of Managua. Three months later those shoes had holes in them, but my legs were strong and sculpted — even better than they had been 20 years ago!

If I can do it, anyone can.

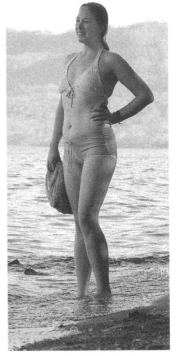

Right: Three months after arriving in Nicaragua I weighed 153 pounds. I maintained that weight for a year and half (until my pregnancy).

Below: After nine months in Nicaragua I returned to Wisconsin. Soon after, I married and became a mom. I'm still learning Spanish, practicing every day with my Guatemalan husband. I modified my diet during my pregnancy and post-partum and am still feeling great.

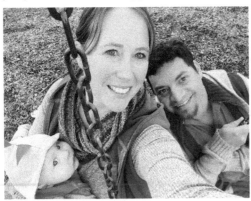

INTRODUCTION

What You'll Find in This Book

FOOD SOBRIETY as a diet and a philosophy is the product of my work in Nicaragua combined with the education and the knowledge I have gleaned from two decades in the healthcare field.

I was inspired to write this book after a life-changing journey through the narrow waist of the Americas. Years ago I began to apply the lessons I learned there to my work in the United States. As my clients shed pounds they asked me for the scientific and philosophical foundations of my unconventional approach. This book was conceived during our conversations.

In **Part One** I discuss my personal weight loss journey while introducing the practices that create both permanent weight loss and build long-term health.

Part Two is a light practical science class that breaks down weight loss into digestible steps, enabling readers to create their own versions of the diet.

Part Three is a stroll through progressive ideas in health, anthropology, and psychology, which come together to form a philosophical foundation that supports sustainable weight loss.

Chapter 15 is inspired by a more recent experience. In 2014 I received a Fulbright Scholar grant to teach nutrition at a university in Nicaragua. I draw from that time for a discussion of the developing world's obesity issues.

Throughout the book Nicaragua is never far away. Every few pages its people and stories pop up to educate, challenge, entertain, and inspire—just as they did for me.

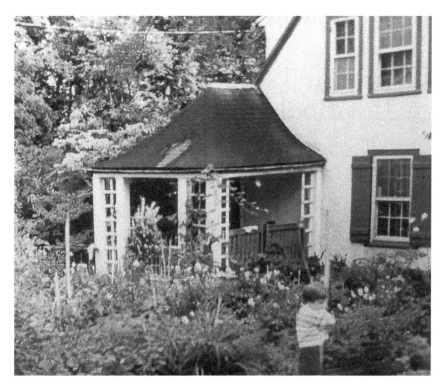

The author planting a stake in the garden, 1979

PREFACE

The String Bean Incident

I noticed that you grow vegetables in the front yard. You may not be aware that our neighborhood is more formal than that.

THE NOTE WAS ANONYMOUS, but we knew the author. The language was delicate, but we knew the meaning. In another time and place a missive of this nature would have sown the seeds of a decade of animosity, but in a town built on diplomacy a different outcome awaited us.

This was early in the 1980s. My family and I lived in Northwest Washington, D.C., in a neighborhood that had rapidly evolved from a comfortable middle-class community to a destination for the prosperous. Our neighbors were lawyers, diplomats, and government officials. Our house was modest but comfortable; our 1972 Dodge Dart an outlier on streets lined with late-model Volvos and BMWs.

If our rusting two-door sedan stood out, then our garden was even more of an aberration. This was no orderly flower garden, but a thousand square feet of productive jungle: raspberry and gooseberry bushes, Hungarian peppers, strawberries, tomatoes, spring onions, chives, Jerusalem artichokes, and salad greens of all kinds. The garden was more than a hobby. My father was a *Washington Post* staff writer and garden columnist who was an early advocate of organic methods. He spent every free moment of daylight weeding, planting, mulching, composting, and harvesting.

Growing up in the 1980s I was keenly aware that my family's front yard wasn't the only thing that marked me as different from my peers. When I was invited to sleepovers at my friends' homes I feasted on steak dinners and sugary breakfast cereals. At home our meals were mostly made with fresh ingredients from our garden or from the vegetable mixes my mother had made and canned. Her packed Mason jars lined the back of every cupboard in the kitchen.

My parents' habits were not a political statement. They were European immigrants who grew up with gardens and home-cooked meals. Continuing to eat this way—and rarely dining at restaurants—had another practical consequence for the family. The substantial savings on food costs meant that they could assist all three of their children in paying for college.

This was in the days before gardening, organics, or even vegetables became at all hip. What was fashionable to our well-heeled neighbors had nothing to do with health. They drank copious cocktails, smoked cigarettes, and ate rich food. The culinary temple of the elite was only a few blocks away, an upscale grocery store called Sutton Place Gourmet. Its broad, immaculate aisles resembled those of a fine furniture store more than a grocery. There was no mention of organic, and there were certainly no bulk bins. "Gourmet" at that time was all about food that was highly flavored, preferably imported, and perfectly packaged: Vermont maple-syrup candies, Alaskan smoked salmon in a "shabby chic" wooden box, ornate tins of Russian caviar, Italian pasta, Spanish olives, Argentine beef, dozens of varieties of French cheese, and a famously large collection of exotically flavored jelly beans, the favorite treat of then-President Reagan.

The health food stores of that era were far from fashionable. Their narrow aisles, haphazard shelves, and uneven fluorescent lighting evoked a thrift store aesthetic, and it was common to find moldy bread and off-tasting yogurt. Expired products weren't surprising—employees were often more interested in reading activist newsletters or planning their next road trip than in taking inventory or stocking shelves.

In the '90s, the gourmet movement, which had once mocked the brown rice crowd, drank the Kool-Aid (*ahem*—the organic smoothie) just in time to capitalize on the growing interest in health food. Chains like Whole Foods and Wild Oats replaced the funky local places, and the corporate mindset turned health food stores into hygienic, efficient, and orderly palaces. This turn of events gave us a gentrified model of health that is just as exclusive as the old Sutton Place Gourmet. Health is now perceived as part of the good life that goes with a big salary—big enough, at least, to buy 90-dollar Lululemon yoga pants and six-dollar loaves of gluten-free bread.

Health has been packaged and sold to us, and it's mostly a rip-off: overpriced, posh grocery stores, organic versions of highly processed junk food, dietary supplements of dubious value, and high-fashion workout clothes.

But let's get back to that note. It was written by our next-door neighbor, an elderly, wealthy patrician woman. Her intent was to notify my parents that in America the land you own and the way you use it is an expression of social class and that we were sending the wrong message. Growing food was something that lower-class people did because they had to scrape together a living. In a wealthy neighborhood, gardens did not include edible plants. The aesthetic ideal was closer to a golf course: meticulously landscaped, with close-shorn grass, borders of flowers, and orderly hedges.

Rather than confront our neighbor or even discuss the matter, my father presented her with bowls of just-picked raspberries and gooseberries. Later, she discovered the superiority of our ripe tomatoes to the ones Sutton Place Gourmet offered. Even though this happened many years ago, my family still remembers that, of all of our diplomatic offerings, she reserved her highest praise for our string beans. This made us all laugh, as they were easy to grow and not particularly unique.

This book is my basket of string beans. It is my invitation to my neighbors to discover a path to health that is inexpensive and simple. Health is a blessing available to all of us.

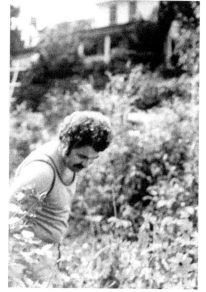

1979: My father, Charles Fenyvesi, in the sprawling, abundant garden that made up our front yard in Washington, D.C. As a teenager, he fought in the failed 1956 Hungarian revolution. Facing a certain prison sentence he escaped Hungary alone and was given political asylum in the U.S. Here he put down roots and, perhaps, planted the seeds of a more peaceful revolution.

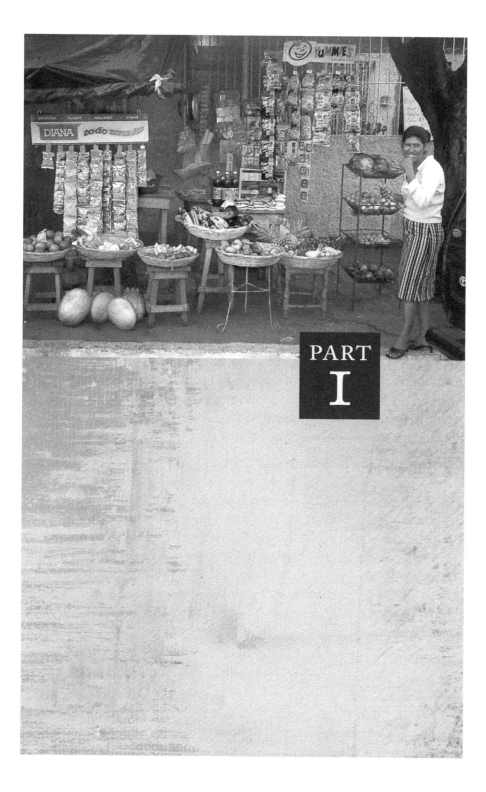

PART
I

CHAPTER 1

Descent Into Gluttony

"Through purity of food comes purity of mind,
through purity of mind comes a steady memory of Truth
and when one gets this memory one becomes free
from all knots of the heart."
CHANDOGYA UPANISHAD, 7.26.2

After nearly a decade of working for pennies at a nutrition supplement company and playing music part time, my tree-hugging Boulder, Colorado, lifestyle came to an abrupt, brokenhearted end. Citing my stubborn lack of ambition, my girlfriend of two years left me. I was lost and depressed. All I could think was that she was right, *she was always right*. My tentative plan was to jump-start my career—and, more importantly, my brain—by getting a master's degree in nutrition. So in 2004, at 32 years old, I went back east and moved in with my parents. I was anxious and miserable, but I had hope that the path ahead would challenge and improve me.

Within a few weeks of my arrival on the East Coast I was taking a heavy course load of prerequisites at Montgomery College in Rockville, Maryland. Attending classes with ambitious young pre-med and pre-pharmacy majors only added to my anxieties. I was part of a study group of five students, all of them on Adderall or Ritalin. They were "study-bots," efficiently downloading information for hours without pause. On rare study breaks they would confidently discuss their meticulously organized goals, all of which included owning a house and being married by 30. While my chemically altered colleagues were focused and driven, I was worried about falling behind.

My anxieties peaked at night when my tossing and turning would twist the bedsheets into a giant cotton pretzel. Sleep-deprived days led me to fall farther behind, and I became mired in a vicious cycle of stress and insomnia. In desperation I, like my drug-addled study group, turned to experimentation: sleeping pills, herbal remedies (valerian and chamomile), Valium, and Benadryl. The "remedies" seemed to help me drift off, but they had me waking up foggy, missing the rejuvenating quality of a good night's sleep. Another unfortunate side effect was that while I had always been a prolific dreamer, my dreams turned into a muddy, incoherent mess when I took meds.

I soon stumbled upon the perfect solution — *drum roll, please!* — food.

When I started school in September I was a trim and fit 140 pounds, thanks to years of hiking every mountain trail in Boulder. In fewer than nine months I gained more than 20 pounds; I lost muscle, and picked up a spare tire, pudgy cheeks, and a new tendency to upset easily and rebound slowly. I was taking courses in organic chemistry, psychology, nutrition, anatomy, and physiology, but I fell into the most common trap my textbooks warned me against: over-indulgence. How could this have happened?

My move home and return to school had prompted me to make *some* healthy changes. In Colorado, I'd lived a life full of measured hedonism balanced by lots of outdoor sports and a wholesome diet. Sober and health oriented throughout the week, I'd spent most Friday and Saturday nights buzzed, either playing bass in my newgrass band or dancing away to a reggae or noodling jam band. Now on the East Coast, I'd made a successful effort to reduce my pot smoking and drinking to once or twice a month. I rewarded myself for my cleaner — or at least more legal — lifestyle with my *new* drug of choice: a tall glass of milk with powdered chocolate and maple syrup. My worries faded with every sip: the 350-plus calories of organic "heroin" floated me off to sleep on a featherbed of sugar and fat.

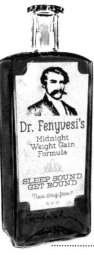

I have always loved sweet flavors. In the past, though, I would save desserts as a way to occasionally reward myself. In the face of my new challenges I lost this discipline, and sweets became an emotional crutch. When I ran out of chocolate and maple syrup, I devolved into a restless bear. After midnight I would stagger out of my cave and go on a quest to satisfy my cravings. Rummaging through cupboards, pushing aside the raisins and rice, spilling the flour and letting the cracker box tumble to the floor, I would gleefully stumble upon some year-old chocolate chips, stale cookies, or my grandmother's diabetic mints. The sweets sent my inner bear into a brief hibernation, a restful sleep valet-parked by a blissful sugar rush.

14 oz. 2% milk	240	*One pound = 3,500 calories, and 3500 ÷ 369 = 9.4*
2 T powdered chocolate	25	So it takes just a little over nine days to gain a pound.
2 T maple syrup	104	**That's 25.5 pounds in eight months.**

369 calories, 11g fat, 44g sugar

My indulgences continued at my part-time job at Whole Foods. I received a hefty employee discount at the deli, and on my shift breaks would enthusiastically order the healthy-looking entrées: salad greens with orange-feta dressing, tofu-veggie skewers with peanut sauce, cucumber-mint quinoa salad, tortilla soup, spinach-ricotta grilled pizza, and turkey burgers on whole wheat buns. Although these dishes were rich in fiber, vitamins, and minerals, they were also calorific, prepared with generous amounts of oil, cheese, dried fruit, nuts, and seeds. In my rush to convert to the emerging trend of healthy fats, I conveniently confused "healthy" with "appropriate for weight loss." Labels blinded me. It wasn't just healthy fats—all my dietary excesses came wrapped up in the feel-good, left-coast packaging: natural, organic, free range, non-GMO, and local. How could any of it cause me harm?

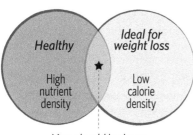

You *should* be here

By the time June rolled around I was a changed man—a soft, buttery 160 pounds. I had completed my prerequisites and drove across country to start graduate school at Bastyr University in Kirkland, Washington. I had never struggled with weight problems before, and my timing couldn't have been worse. Bastyr, a place dominated by beautiful, intelligent women, should have been heaven for me. Sadly, the Bastyr women were immune to my chubby, insecure charm. The rejections, along with the weight of more student loans and the daunting academic workload, only served to solidify my new bad habits.

Like a disgruntled, overworked waiter I would take "smoke breaks" from the library. My cigarettes were energy bars, nuts, and smoothies. The treats relaxed me and were a reward for finishing a chapter, a paper, or a project. I often capped all-night study sessions with dinners at a nearby Indian restaurant where every meal was soaked in saffron-scented butter. All my anxiety and stress felt manageable when I ate. A full belly was an air bag for the car crashes of daily life.

I convinced myself that I wasn't turning into a glutton. I was just transforming into a "foodie," a hip connoisseur who selects food for its pedigree—taking origin, production method, and environmental impact into account. These are important considerations; we should all take responsibility for the impact of our decisions. However, it is all too easy to confuse doing a good deed for the environment with consuming what is appropriate for our personal health goals.

If the environmental imperative happened to fail, then I could always find a handy nutritional excuse for every rich choice: olive oil is good for the heart, wild salmon has omega-3 fatty acids, almonds have magnesium, red wine has resveratrol, and unpasteurized goat cheese has probiotics. With everyone rushing to certify chocolate for its medicinal properties, I was not to be left behind. My new therapy for sleepless nights was dark chocolate slathered in almond butter (300-plus calories per "session"). The intense mix of fat and sugar melted my tension and soothed my nerves with pharmaceutical potency, but filled my stomach for all of an hour.

I morphed into a docile, tubby cat content to waddle over to a bowl of warm milk whenever a new challenge stressed me. My frequent feedings affected more than my weight. For the first time in my life my digestion was so consistently off it became a daily hassle. It is hard to pay attention in class when your stomach gurgles or when you feel bloated and gassy. Some days I was constipated and other days I had four bowel movements before lunch. One naturopathic physician diagnosed me with irritable bowel syndrome and another said I had Crohn's disease. My digestion, energy, and emotional stability were all slipping down a greasy, sugary slope.

By the time I finished my first year of graduate school, I weighed 170 pounds. The irony of gaining weight while studying nutrition failed to amuse me. Even odder was that I had spent years playing in bands, surrounded by hedonism,

Surprised? Kale chips have more nutrients, but when you're trying to lose weight they're as poor a choice as other typical snack foods.

Nutrition Facts	
Serving Size 1 oz.	
Servings per container 16	
Amount Per Serving	
Calories 140 Calories from Fat 70	
	% Daily Value*
Total Fat 8g	12%
Saturated Fat 1g	6%
Trans Fat 0g	0%
Cholesterol 0mg	0%
Sodium 210mg	9%
Total Carbohydrate 16g	5%
Dietary Fiber 3g	4%
Sugars 5g	0%
Protein 2g	4%
Vitamin A 2% Calcium 6%	

Nacho Cheese Chips BAM!

Kale Chips HEALTH EXPLOSION!

Nutrition Facts	
Serving Size 1 oz.	
Servings per container 16	
Amount Per Serving	
Calories 150 Calories from Fat 80	
	% Daily Value*
Total Fat 9g	14%
Saturated Fat 1g	5%
Trans Fat 0g	0%
Cholesterol 0mg	0%
Sodium 220mg	9%
Total Carbohydrate 11g	4%
Dietary Fiber 3g	5%
Sugars 4g	0%
Protein 6g	4%
Vitamin A 2% Vitamin C 10%	
Calcium 15% Iron 10%	

and despite being offered all sorts of free alcohol and drugs I never developed anything close to an addiction. Now I was laid low by kale chips, dark chocolate, toasted almonds, and smoothies. Trying to find the silver lining, I thought: How can I counsel overweight patients if I have never grappled with the issue myself? How can I appreciate good health without having struggled first? Like countless others, I unwittingly performed a science experiment on myself.

My Path to Food Sobriety

I've always been an experimenter. Over the past 20 years I studied and enthusiastically tried dozens of dietary approaches, including raw, vegetarian, vegan, orthorexic, fasting, cleanses, Atkins, Paleo, Mediterranean, South Beach, high protein, and good old American overindulgence (the "greenwashed" version I described in the past few pages). While each approach yielded insights, the

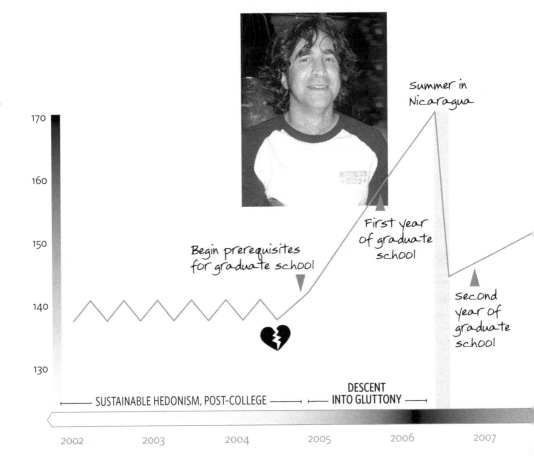

most valuable came from my experiences in Nicaragua and from applying those lessons to my work with clients in the United States.

Most of us share a craving for delicious, high-calorie food. Clearly I love everything bad for me: sweets, rich foods, alcohol, and the feeling of being stuffed silly. While I still recognize the appeal of these experiences, I am no longer addicted to them. Over the past few years my weight has dropped from an all-time high of 170 pounds to 135, my waist from 35 inches to 30, and my body fat from 25 percent to less than 15. On a lightly-built 5'6" frame, losing 35 pounds was a considerable success. It was one-fifth of my body weight, the equivalent of taking off a backpack with four-and-a-half gallons of water in it. Without that extra weight to lug around, I no longer have knee pain, back pain, digestive problems, or sore feet. My energy and self-confidence are higher while my stress level has diminished.

Outlining my weight history helped me understand influential turning points. This exercise has also proven revealing for many of my clients. I recommend sketching your own past, as well as how you envision a better future.

Returned to Nicaragua, recreated the diet, and began this book. Lost 20 lbs. more.

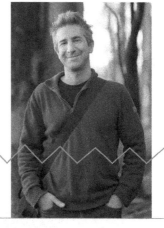

The 10 lbs that returned during my second year of grad school stuck around for the next three years.

2008   2009   2010   2011   2012   2013   2014   2015   2016   2017

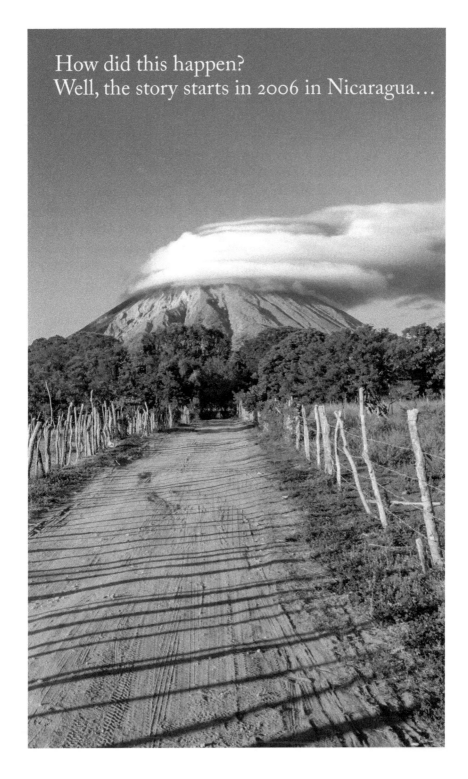

How did this happen?
Well, the story starts in 2006 in Nicaragua…

CHAPTER 2

From Shipwreck to Sobriety

"No man can learn what he has not preparation for learning, however near to his eyes is the object. A chemist may tell his most precious secrets to a carpenter, and he shall be never the wiser — the secrets he would not utter to a chemist for an estate. God screens us evermore from premature ideas. Our eyes are holden that we cannot see things that stare us in the face, until the hour arrives when the mind is ripened; then we behold them, and the time when we saw them not is like a dream."

RALPH WALDO EMERSON, *SELECTED ESSAYS, LECTURES, AND POEMS*

IN THE SUMMER OF 2006 I RECEIVED A SMALL RESEARCH GRANT from my graduate school to study healthcare in Nicaragua. For three months I lived in the hot, grubby, sprawling capital that is Managua, and traveled the country interviewing doctors, nutritionists, public health officials, traditional healers, herbalists, cooks, restaurant owners, and others about diet and healthcare. Without exception I found Nicaraguans to be inviting, patient, and friendly. Not only were they more than willing to sit for long interviews, but I was often invited to collaborate on projects, to visit clinics, and to eat homemade meals with their families.

When I interviewed people in the capital, small cities, and the more accessible parts of the countryside, I found that North American ideas about diet were increasingly influential. People strongly preferred foods that had come to Nicaragua in the second half of the 20th century: pasta, bread, soda, sweets, and fried food. They also ate as much meat, cheese, and processed food as they could afford.

When I visited more remote communities—those without electricity, phone lines, or paved roads—I found diets limited to a dozen or so local crops. In 2006 the people in those communities were, in general, healthier, with far lower rates of chronic disease and obesity than their urban counterparts.* Although they enjoyed rich foods only on special occasions, they didn't express strong cravings or desires for those treats. Instead, they expressed satisfaction

---

* In the last decade, as urban food habits have spread, this is no longer true.

with their diet and clearly felt a deep connection to their staple foods. They benefited from and enjoyed simple and repetitive diets (as have thousands of other traditional communities), needing to make only a fraction of the decisions about food that Americans do.

Researching the impact of variety and surplus on dietary decisions, Cornell University professor Brian Wansink calculated that the average American makes approximately 226 decisions about food a day, while obese people make well over 300 decisions.[1] Wansink's study showed that as access to quantity and variety of food increases, consumption rises proportionally. The external factors — the variety and abundance — are the stimuli that reliably predict how much people eat, while the internal factors — hunger and biological needs — have surprisingly little influence.

In the Western world we only have to go back three or four generations to find a time when our daily decisions about food amounted to a few dozen. Then, we made just a handful of decisions about diet. We ate what was in season and foods that could be stored without refrigeration. Prior to the development of agriculture we ate anything that we could find, forage, or scavenge. The whole earth was our grocery store, and we walked its aisles pulling down leaves, digging up roots, and stalking prey.

....

Platos Típicos. In Nicaraguan cities, where salaries are higher, people can afford to eat more animal products and the vegetable oil in which to fry them. In the poorest parts of the countryside people used to eat only what they could grow — beans, corn, and produce. In the past decade, however, oil, sugar, animal products, and processed foods have become widespread.

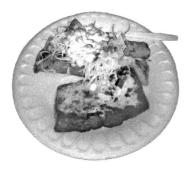

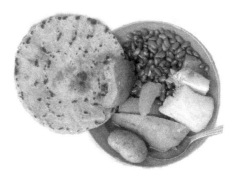

Deep-fried cheese and deep-fried beef tacos with sour cream and a sprinkling of cabbage salad

Beans, boiled vegetables, and a corn tortilla

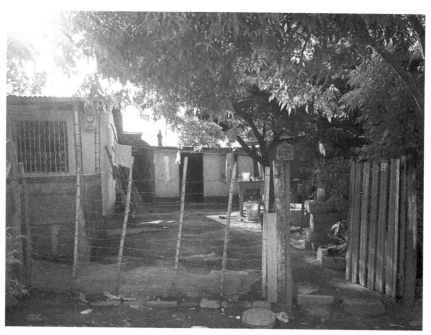

A typical home on the street where I lived. *(Barrio Edgar Munguia, Managua)*

The Time-Travel Chronicles of Beneficial Deprivations

My sleep was interrupted by a melodic voice. I rubbed my eyes and looked out my window to see a donkey-drawn wooden cart laden with a pyramid of watermelons. A young boy perched atop the pyramid called out prices as the donkey's hooves kicked up dust from the road.

I was on a tight budget. My monthly rent in Managua was 80 dollars and my daily budget varied between five and 10 dollars. I rented a room in the modest home of a kind couple. When showing me their house for the first time they proudly pointed out their new linoleum floor. Most homes had dirt floors, corrugated tin roofs, and small yards enclosed by dilapidated sheet metal topped with embedded broken glass to deter thieves.

I saved on meals by eating at a neighborhood *fritanga* (food stand—literally, "frying place"), a plywood cabana the size of a VW van, with a few plastic chairs. Nicaraguan fritangas offer beans, white rice, plantains, tortillas, chicken, beef, and cheese. Most everything is fried in vegetable oil, which is reused all day long as it is quite expensive by local standards. The only vegetable is diced cabbage soaked in vinegar.

I ate only fritanga food my first week in the country. As a result, my stomach hurt, my face was breaking out, and I could feel myself getting heavier. Worst of all, I started every meal bitterly mumbling, "If it's bad for me it should at least *taste* good." My bourgeois palate was repulsed by all of it, but the funky grease oozing off every plate was just too much. I was relieved when I stumbled upon a unique fritanga a few blocks from my barrio. Its owner had spent years working with a health-oriented nonprofit project in the 1980s and she tried her best to stick to those ideals. She didn't fry her food, and a plate of brown rice, beans, and steamed vegetables or cabbage salad ran less than a dollar. I ate that dish (with slight variations) two to three times a day all summer. I also ate soft-boiled eggs most mornings and had fresh fruit several times a day.

While I was grateful to have a healthy option, the food hardly tasted better and my dietary transition was difficult. I cursed myself for not saving more money over the years. If I had just set aside a thousand dollars, I could have spared myself this austere diet. There were no herbs or spices. The beans tasted like my sweat-soaked shirt, and the rice was dry—undercooked just enough to be tough and chewy. I called it "rice jerky." The vegetables were a colorless, forgettable lot, steamed as soft as baby food. Not only was it flavorless, this food didn't *do* anything for me. There was no pick-me-up from sugar, no relaxing fat buzz, and (because of my budget) no escape. Few foreign foods were available in Nicaragua, and those that were imported (packaged, frozen, and canned) were twice as expensive as in the States. My diet consisted of whatever was locally available and in season, fewer than a dozen or so fruits and vegetables at one time.

I came to the depressing realization that I had lost my favorite coping mechanism. In the States when I was frustrated I used to grab what I thought of as healthy pick-me-ups: trail mix, protein bars, a smoothie, a bran muffin, or kale chips. They were edible therapy: they made me forget how tired I was, how much my knees hurt, or how far behind I was in an endless series of obligations. All the little smoke alarms that my body was emitting were efficiently smothered by excess fat and sugar. In Nicaragua I couldn't bring myself to indulge in the local equivalents—fried food and the sweets sold in barrio shops: peanuts covered in salt and sugar; cheap, gooey chocolate that was half hydrogenated vegetable oil; and ice cream with a peculiar sandy texture (frequent power outages meant that the texture of frozen foods was notoriously unpredictable). Without my hippie gourmet delicacies to reach for, I never escaped reality.

My cravings intensified. Potent flavors lingered in my memory. I dreamed of Muenster cheese, rye bread, buttery Ritz crackers, granola, turkey bacon, smoked salmon, anchovies, LARA bars, kombucha, chocolate, herbal teas, pizza, my mom's ratatouille, my grandmother's goulash, cream of tomato soup, almonds, sesame oil, olive oil, my beloved saag paneer, and toast with butter and honey. But, like a marooned sailor, I was out of luck—or so I thought. Then, about a month into my gastronomic shipwreck, an unexpected metamorphosis began.

The Revelation

The first hint of improvement occurred with the beans. I started to detect nutty, dark, and creamy tastes. The new flavors were faint at first but they grew stronger. I was experiencing increasing excitement about *beans*—this was truly a first! Next, the vinegar-soaked cabbage piqued my interest. Its mix of crunchy and sour offered a refreshing, perky contrast that was like a cold shower for my long hung-over taste buds. Even the rice began to taste good—sweet and light. I began to notice subtle elements of the meal: how the food was arranged, the slight variations in the shape and size of the grains, how thinly or thickly sliced the cabbage was, and how hot the meal was served.

I made an effort to learn about the local vegetables—their names and where they were grown. Nicaragua has two distinct seasons, one wet and the other dry. Since my trip started in the dry season and ended in the wet one I became familiar with the crops planted and harvested in each. I became fond of a particular squash called chayote, which grows on long vines and looks like a pear. When steamed, its texture reminded me of butter. Maybe it was just that I hadn't had any butter in months. Had I forgotten the flavor? The explanation hardly matters—I was just happy to be enjoying food again. Later I noticed the underlying acidity in tropical fruits, and the many textures of the diverse varieties of mango. My curiosity led to questions for my curbside fruit vendors: "Where is the fruit from today? Is it *dulce* (sweet) or *agrio* (sour)?" Like slowly taking interest in someone you once thought was dull, learning a food's background story makes it more appealing and even affects how you perceive its taste.

My sense of taste wasn't the only sense becoming finely tuned. When I first got to Nicaragua I categorized all the music I was hearing as "Latin music." As my ears became attuned to the sounds, I picked up that *salsa* has a "1-2-3, 1-2" rhythm, that *cumbia* focuses on drums and *claves*, that *merengue* is fast and has a ¾ beat, and that *bachata* is romantic and slow, with blissful vocals.

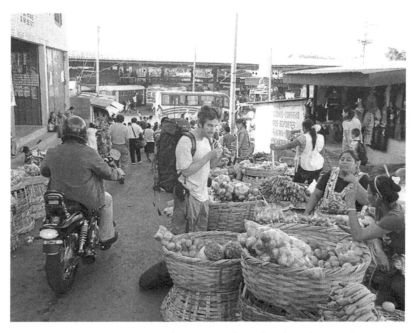

Once I began enjoying my meals, I ventured into local markets with an open mind, a far more forgiving palate, and a head full of questions for the vendors.
(Mercado Israel Lewites, Managua)

It helped that I was adopting a Nicaraguan attitude toward mealtimes, and taking it slow. When you spend longer chewing, your tongue has more time to pick up subtler flavors. It became a daily source of wonder that the meals that once bored me to tears were now so satisfying. While it is our nature to evaluate everything comparatively, our demanding perspective fades as variety diminishes. What remains is simple satisfaction, like that of an animal eating.

The diet I'd adopted as a financial necessity had developed into a spiritual discipline and was yielding tangible results. It happened quietly. After about a month I noticed that my clothes were getting very loose. Following a rough week or two of adjustment, my digestive system began to work perfectly for the first time in years. I could set my watch to my swift and effortless bathroom breaks. The predictability of the meals was like a holiday for my intestines. ("Beans, corn, and veggies again? No problem—we've got this down!") It made me wonder if our digestive tracts are actually built to handle the wide variety inherent in modern diets. My temperament and energy levels steadied, my cravings faded, and the restless honey-seeking bear went into hibernation.

I was developing a new relationship with food that in turn was nourishing me in ways I had never imagined possible.

Skeptics might argue that those benefits were a result of the excitement of overseas travel. As this was my second extended stay in Nicaragua, I had a basis for comparison. During my first trip in 2002 (a three-month-long volunteer project), my energy and mood were unaffected and I had many digestive complaints. At that time I had a larger budget and ate at middle-class restaurants that served the usual assortment of cheeses, meats, oils, nuts, sweets, and juices.

These truths—the flexible nature of taste (or desire) and the healing qualities of an ascetic diet—could have never revealed themselves at home, in a high-income country. In a wealthy society the perpetual abundance and broad variety of foods keep our taste buds so overstimulated that a simple diet feels like a punishment. I had to go to the second-poorest country in the Western Hemisphere to develop my new connection with food. Since most people aren't dying to go to Nicaragua to live on rice, beans, and cabbage, I wrote this book to guide readers in creating their own transformative experience, one that works with a variety of food and dietary approaches.

That summer in Nicaragua I gained perspective and I lost 25 pounds. The weight loss came as a direct result of my diet. It was not connected to my physical activity, which declined. The barrio I lived in had no trash service, and garbage was burned in little piles on the sidewalk. It's hard to jog or play soccer while breathing in fumes of burning plastic. The moist, tropical heat dampened my drive as well. Most days were well over 90 degrees Fahrenheit, and at night only my fan on high speed allowed me to drift to sleep. Whether I remained sleeping a few hours later was an iffy proposition—crowing roosters and fan-stopping power outages were a near-nightly experience. The drains on my energy meant that my sole regular exercise besides walking was halfhearted attempts at salsa dancing and some equally listless weight lifting. The other factor affecting my weight loss was a decreased stress level. I was enjoying my project, making friends, and living life at a fairly relaxed pace.

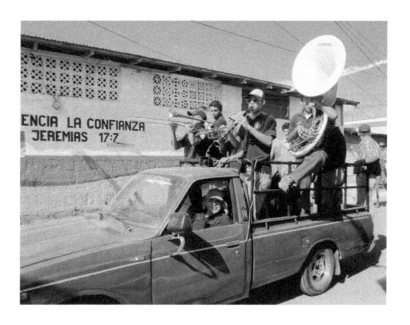

The Nicaraguan Character

There is no better place to learn the
art of food sobriety than Nicaragua.

Nicas, as they like to be called, are by necessity experts at enjoying a
spartan life. In Nicaragua nothing is certain. The long history of corrupt
and inept governments has produced countless scandals, revolutions,
and bloody repressions that are matched by a geography that regularly
produces earthquakes, floods, and volcanic eruptions. All of this un-
certainty has built a national personality with an ingenious ability to
produce joy from the limited resources available. Nicas also love to play.
They sing while doing dishes, turn tin cans into soccer balls, spin engaging stories, recite poems, and are always ready to dance.

Diet's Daily Effect on Energy and Mood

In Nicaragua I realized that whether I had a great day or a lousy day had nothing to do with what I ate. How could it? My meals varied little from day to day. My mood and energy levels became liberated from my diet. The fog of diet-induced sensations lifted, and the nature of my emotions—why and how they originated—came into focus. It is not that I entered a state of permanent bliss. I had moments of loneliness, self-pity, boredom, and fear. The difference was that I could trace the roots of my emotions to their source.

The mini benders on caffeine, sweets, and rich food that would elicit animated, contented conversations disappeared along with their flip side: the cranky, low-energy lulls that followed. I was rarely caught off guard by a sudden sinking feeling, frustration from unfulfilled cravings, or guilt from overindulgence. My natural cues for hunger, sleep, relaxation, happiness, and social contact felt more genuine and predictable. The experience made me wonder if we manipulate our feelings so often that we end up needing professional help to connect to our emotions.

....

When people ask, "How was your day?" if your response goes beyond small talk, you are likely to report on a meal you ate. "I had a great day, had burgers and fries with Trey and Mike." Or "Hectic day! I ate greasy Chinese takeout in my car." Perhaps you had an invigorating Mediterranean lunch with a friend and a productive afternoon, or you had a rushed pizza dinner and felt cranky and lethargic all evening. *What and how you eat affects your day and becomes part of the story of your life.*

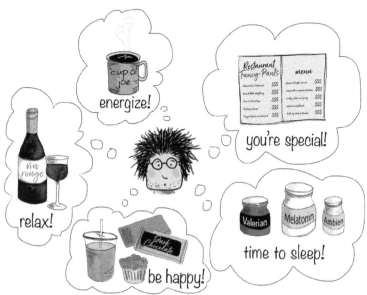

I also felt liberated from my North American fixation on food. It was a relief that I rarely thought about my meals outside of mealtimes. The quality of my day depended on progress in my research, interaction with friends and strangers, the book I was reading, the salsa class I took, and the Spanish words I learned. My mental acuity strengthened and I became more focused on the activities of life — *doing* and not just *consuming*. I stopped even thinking about my diet. It became like sleep, something I loved and needed, but that required no thought. Because my repetitive meals provided only minimal distraction, I felt more engaged by the company with whom I shared my meals. Conversations became the spice of mealtimes.

A Twist at the End

During the last two weeks of my three-month stay in Nicaragua, my old friend Mark visited me. A hardworking American on vacation, Mark wanted no part of my peasant-style meals. To accommodate him, I took him to "fancy" Nicaraguan restaurants. We went out the first night to a five- to ten-dollar-a-plate restaurant. In 2006 five dollars was more than the average daily salary in Managua. Locals celebrate wedding anniversaries, retirement parties, and birthdays in places like this. That first night we strolled in and ate with the high end of Nicaraguan society. We had a large, rich meal of steak, potatoes, rice, cheese, and fresh-squeezed fruit juice.

My taste buds were overwhelmed by the caloric blitz. Every bite was a whirlwind of salt, herbs, meaty juices, and butter. The mouthwatering flavors brought me back to a life lived in another time and place. My mind drifted to a Passover at my parents' farm in Maryland and a Thanksgiving at my brother's home in Connecticut, and then my thoughts really took flight. Was I a feasting baron in the feudal Hungary of my ancestors? Or maybe I was just the peasant cook in the baron's kitchen? The meal was sending my grease-soaked brain off into a fantasy world. Baron, cook, or graduate student, it hardly mattered. The food was so engaging that it was hard to even pay attention to the conversation with my old friend. (*"Hey — keep it down, buddy! I'm traveling through time with the steak and potatoes!"*)

As upscale as the ambiance of the restaurant was, the quality of the food was, as Mark reminded me, run of the mill. Mark rated it a slight cut below Olive Garden or TGIFridays. As much as I enjoyed the meal, the next day I had no desire to return to that style of eating. We went out to eat several times a day during Mark's week-long stay. I found myself, to the waiters' befuddlement, ordering a cup of beans, a bowl of steamed vegetables, and a few tortillas or ears of steamed corn. The indulgence had been exciting and enjoyable, but I felt happy returning to the basic flavors I had recently embraced. Like a well-worn pair of jeans, they felt just right.

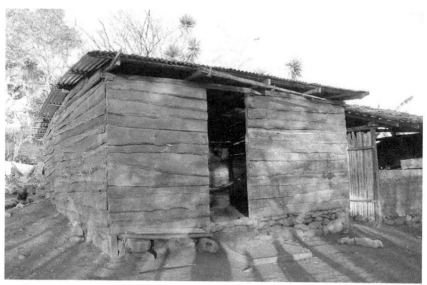

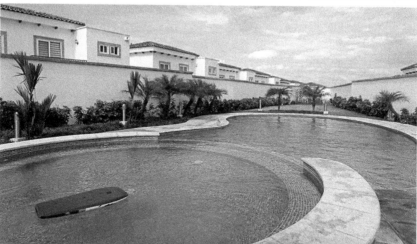

The class disparity in Nicaragua is vast. The average Nicaraguan makes less than 10 dollars a day and has an education equivalent to the sixth grade in the U.S. In contrast, those in the upper echelon live like royalty. They attend private universities in the U.S. and Europe and take weekend shopping trips to Miami, Houston, and Los Angeles. Their homes are massive fortresses with high walls and private security, maintained by housekeepers, nannies, and gardeners.

(top: Los Pinares; bottom: Managua)

A Forkful of History

As Mark and I waited for our dinner we took in an entertaining scene at the table next to us. It looked like the high life: a group of boisterous, expensively dressed older gentlemen at a beautifully set table piled high with gourmet food and plenty of alcohol.

The men burst into song several times. The first was a classic I had heard a few times: "Managua, Nicaragua Donde Yo Me Enamore" (Managua, Nicaragua Where I Fell in Love), a sweet folk song about love. The next had a more militant feel. I could make out some of the lyrics, something about soldiers, honor, and freedom. Not wanting to interrupt the partying neighbors, I asked our waiter, "Do you know what song this is?"

The waiter grimaced, "Oh, this is 'Hermosa Soberana Nicaragua'" (Beautiful Sovereign Nicaragua). Curiosity piqued, I pressed on. "It sounds like a patriotic song. Is it about the revolution?"

"No, no," the waiter replied. "It is a pre-revolution song, actually almost like a Somoza anthem."

"They are pro-Somoza?"

"Yes, it is a reunion of former Somoza associates."

"Really? I can't believe it."

He smiled and said, "Yes, look at how luxuriously they dine."

Because Nicaraguans love talking about politics and history, I knew it was a rarity to run into Somoza loyalists. The 43-year reign of the Somoza family exacerbated inequality by monopolizing the country's resources and stealing land to give to supporters; opposition was suppressed with a brutal police force.

The societal inequity was also reflected in the diet. During the Somoza era the poor majority ate the traditional diet (the one I grew to love), while the wealthy minority ate the kind of rich, Western-influenced fare the upscale restaurant served. The dietary divide peaked in the years after a devastating 1972 earthquake. As the populace suffered through food shortages, the Somozas and their supporters embezzled international relief funds and sold much of the foreign food aid in the black market. The corruption was a tipping point in the public support of Somoza; by the end of the decade a revolution dispatched the Somozas.

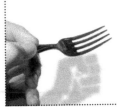

While disparities still characterize Nicaragua, the decades that followed the revolution have seen a more equitable distribution of some resources, including food. This history occasionally came up during my dietary surveys; some of my subjects viewed the lack of food shortages and the availability of modern foods as evidence of the gains of the revolution.

The Passage Back to Complexity

I returned home from Nicaragua and quickly found myself in familiar environs: the fifth-floor dormitory at Bastyr. Eager to show off my disappearing butter belly, I headed straight to where the beautiful women of Bastyr gathered: the communal kitchen. During the first few weeks of school I would sit down every few evenings as they tuned into the consensus favorite, The Food Network. I was reintroduced to Rachel Ray and Emeril and the various shows about the history of Hershey, Twinkies, sausage, or soda. In the past I would easily tune out the TV just to be around this lively group. However, something had changed—and I *couldn't* tune it out.

I was struck by not only by the intensity of the focus on food, but by the kinds of foods that were the subject: program after program displayed its reverence for man-made food creations. After three months of being not just contented with a spartan diet, but healed by it, I was irritated to see such complex and highly refined foods glorified like celebrities. Where were the programs on wholesome foods? There was never anything on whole foods like split peas, peppers, or potatoes.

The cooking shows seemed ridiculous, with their long lists of ingredients, their many kitchen gadgets, and the endless steps and procedures needed to make dishes. Who has an hour to prepare dinner? Who wants to spend 50 dollars on ingredients? These shows were Martha Stewart fantasies.

The glorification of excess and the overcomplication of how and what to eat didn't stop at the Food Network. I saw it everywhere. Every third conversation was about food—what to eat, the new "it" restaurant, what the hot new food trends were, how to make this or that dish, how bad the customer service at this bistro was, or how exotic the ambiance at such-and-such cafe was. Food had become the new weather. It was the topic of default when no shared interests could be found, the non-controversial filler to augment awkward moments of silence. The conversation now sounded neurotic and trivial to me. What an ironic development—I had always been fascinated by people's dietary choices.

In rural Nicaragua the topic of food doesn't come up naturally, and people aren't inclined to rank food preferences. The daily differences are so minor that discussing them seems pointless. It is like asking Americans if they prefer gasoline from Shell or Exxon. In most of Nicaragua people don't even vary the type of beans or rice they eat. Despite this, the most common comment

I heard was that they love their diet and have never had any conflict or confusion over what to eat. Regardless of their own responses, my interview subjects were surprised about my fixation on diet and were always eager to steer the conversation back to subjects that they were passionate about: family, philosophy, agriculture, religion, music, politics, and jokes—many, many jokes.

Organizing foods into a hierarchy of quality and pleasure is unique to the developed world, to high-income countries. In the developing world all food is pleasure and diet is valued for sustenance, not for its ability to dazzle or soothe. Satisfaction comes from the communal experience, the relaxation, the break from work, and the conversation.[2] I bring this philosophy to Food Sobriety. *You do not need to drop your passion for food;* rather, you benefit from cultivating a primal love of all nourishing food.

I came to two conclusions after those first weeks back at Bastyr. One, being around the women wasn't worth having to sit through the Food Network. Two, we need to move past our food obsession. For nearly our entire history we have been haunted by the inability to have a consistent and plentiful food supply. We now have the most abundant and diverse food supply in history, yet we never stop discussing how to get more pleasure from eating. In our drive to squeeze more out of the culinary experience we have exchanged our past, diseases of scarcity, for the present epidemic of chronic disease.[3]

This problem can be seen as a pendulum swinging between two extremes: on one end of the arc scarcity, and on the other, overconsumption. The answer lies in the middle, where there is balance. The shortages and anxieties of the past, as well as the gluttony and disease of the present, are left behind for the future: Food Sobriety.

NOTES

1   Brian Wansink and Jeffery Sobal, "Mindless eating. The 200 daily food decisions we overlook." *Environment and Behaviour* 39 (2007), 106-123. Wansink is a professor and director of the Cornell University Food and Brand Lab. He is a leading expert in changing eating behavior using principles of behavioral science.

2   Léonie N. Dapi, Cécile Omoloko, et al. "'I eat to be happy, to be strong, and to live.' Perceptions of Rural and Urban adolescents in Cameroon, Africa." *J Nutr Educ Behav* 39(6), 320-6.

3   *Diseases of scarcity/insufficient nutrients* generally occur against our will (except in the case of hunger strikes or intentional fasting) or because of a lack of knowledge. Occasionally genetics plays a role. These diseases include kwashiorkor, marasmus, xerophthalmia, beriberi, pellagra, scurvy, rickets, goiter, anemia, failure to thrive, and stunted growth. *Chronic diseases* come from lifestyle choices such as tobacco/drug/alcohol use, lack of physical activity, chronic stress, and poor eating habits. They include cardiovascular diseases such as heart attacks and stroke, some cancers, diabetes, and oral health problems.

4   *(see p. 23)* Danny Fenyvesi, "Nicaragua Solar," *Home Power*, Issue 97. October/November 2003, 58.

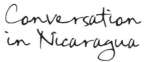

Conversation in Nicaragua

On my first trip to Nicaragua I spent several months volunteering with Grupo Fenix, a nonprofit group that works with solar ovens. These ovens are made from materials such as wood, cardboard, aluminum foil, and Plexiglas. They are inexpensive to build and use no fuel. They create heat by trapping sunlight in an insulated box. Many organizations promote their use to reduce fuel costs, decrease air pollution (and the associated lung and eye damage caused by cooking over wood fires), and reduce deforestation caused by gathering firewood for cooking. On one of our expeditions we traveled to a remote mountain village named Las Pintadas ("The Paintings," after ancient petroglyphs found on nearby rocks). Las Pintadas had no running water, electricity, or plumbing. I wrote about the experience for *Home Power* magazine.[4]

On my first night there I sat with an inquisitive group of locals, most of whom had never met, or even seen, a gringo. They had a crumpled old map of the world on the wall and wanted me to explain where I lived. I pointed to San Francisco and they asked many questions, such as: "Is the fishing good? Does it snow a lot? How many kilometers is it to walk to your parents'?" I pointed to Maryland and explained that my parents lived there. A roomful of eyes studied the vast expanse between the two cities and there was an uncomfortable silence. Finally someone spoke up: "Was your father a drunk?" Then another voice: "Was there a flood?" One more voice replied, "Of course you moved because there were no jobs in Maryland." I explained that distance between family members is common in the States, and my answer led to a night full of questions and discussions about geography, culture, and the meaning of family. I was struck by the intense curiosity about the world that is unique to people who will never have the means to see it.

PART
2

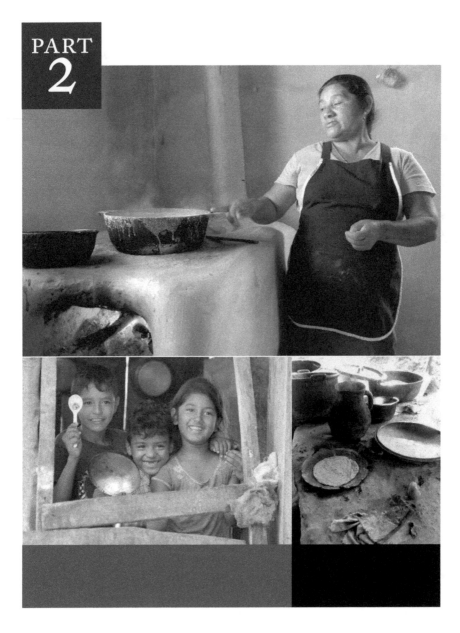

CHAPTER 3

The Food Sobriety Diet

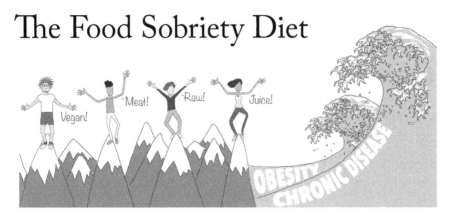

LIKE POLITICIANS ON THE CAMPAIGN TRAIL, diet gurus preach with unfettered optimism about the one true path (theirs!) that leads to the pinnacle. Their passion and their ideas can be captivating. Some of their dietary philosophies even include appeals to admirable ecological and animal-rights goals. Still—whether you're listening to the vegetarian activist, the Paleo pusher, the raw foods preacher, the juicer, or the qualitarian—all of these approaches are overly simplistic.

Again like politicians, diet gurus vie for your support with the promise of easy, one-size-fits-all solutions. **There is no single solution.** Humans are diverse, with varying genetics, lifestyles, medical histories, desires, beliefs, and customs. A healthcare professional promoting rigid dietary dogma like "high protein" and "low carb" is akin to a physicist proclaiming "Neutrons are junk, only electrons matter." Atoms need protons, electrons, and neutrons; humans need proteins, carbohydrates, and fats.

You can have long-term success with a variety of dietary paths as long as you keep three principles in mind. All diets must:

1 Produce a calorie deficit

2 Create satiety

3 Provide sufficient daily nutrients for health: at minimum, 1,200 calories, 50 grams of protein, 130 grams of carbohydrate, 25 grams of fiber, and 10 to 20 grams of essential fatty acids.

The term **qualitarian** was popularized by dietitian Ashley Koff. It refers to choosing unprocessed organic foods: no hormones, GMOs, or unethical practices (like raising chickens without sunlight or space for natural movement).

Everything beyond the minimums is a choice. You might lose weight on a low- or moderate-fat diet, a high-protein diet, or a diet that just meets the minimum requirements. The same applies to carbohydrates: some people do well with a diet that is mostly carbohydrates, while others thrive hovering over the minimum.

Successful diets also come in a variety of philosophical frameworks: vegetarian, carnivore, whole foods, even highly processed. Your goal is not to adapt to someone else's dietary ideal — the follow-the-leader concept — but to craft a diet that you can believe in.

Consider the rest of the chapter a road map that will help you to be your own diet guru. The guidelines, and the sample menus that follow, are potent. Some of you won't have to be quite as strict to realize your goals and many will want to experiment with variations. I encourage this — tailor the diet to best fit your needs.

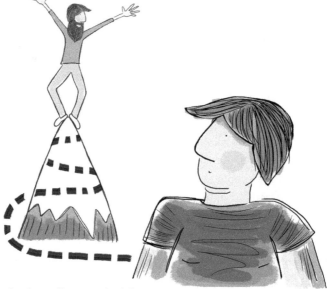

Some notes about the three dietary principles:
- **Be careful with your calorie deficit and satiety.** If your calorie deficit is too large — for instance, if you are burning over 3,000 calories a day but are taking in fewer than 1,200 calories — your metabolism will eventually slow. You'll feel sluggish and cranky, weight loss will stop, and you'll feel a constant, gnawing hunger. *The most sustainable long-term diets have deficits between 100 and 500 calories,* though many people do well for shorter intervals with deficits over 1,000 calories.
- **Nutrient recommendations** are generally agreed-upon minimums established by the U.S. government and research institutions to avoid deficiencies and maintain health. Because lifestyles, body types, and genetics differ these numbers will vary by individual. The details of nutrient needs and options are covered in Chapters 5–8.

The Sober Plate

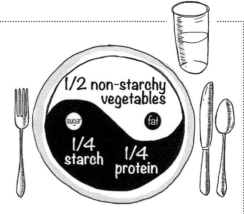

In an age of complexity,
a diet of simplicity

The Food Sobriety diet is based on mainstream science. Its origin is in the Plate Method, developed decades ago as a blood sugar management tool for diabetics.

I taught the Plate Method in public health clinics because it was a simple visual tool that worked well. As I tracked my patients' diets and weight I noticed a few trends that correlated with weight loss and a few with weight gain. That information inspired me to research ways to overhaul the Plate Method to maximize weight loss. I tested my adjustments to the diet with my patients, and found that those who followed the diet were thrilled with the results.

While there are many versions of the Plate Method in use, few distinguish between starchy and fibrous vegetables. Most do not even separate fruits and vegetables, simply declaring that half the plate can be any mix of the two. The traditional Plate Methods include generous amounts of dairy and don't account for the degree of processing in the food, the fiber content, or the fat content. I have made all these and more modifications to my overhauled Plate Method, which I call the **Sober Plate.**

3 The Sober Plate's mantra is three. There are three stages to this program, three steps in each stage, three meals a day, up to three snacks, and most importantly, three parts to every meal:

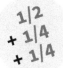

For every meal you eat, imagine dividing your plate in half, then dividing one side in half again. The large section is for vegetables. The other two are evenly divided between starches and proteins, with low- and nonfat dairy counting as a protein.

You might wonder if this is a radical diet that will work your intestines like cherry soda and funnel cake before a roller coaster ride. The truth is, if you made the transition to this diet all at once you would be in discomfort. **I advise building up to this diet using the three-stage approach described on page 30.**

Food Sobriety: Broad Strokes and Nuances

1   The Sober Plate emphasizes dietary balance and flexibility.

Another way to think of the Sober Plate is that it contains two parts, a heavy part (starch and protein) and a light part (veggies). Your plate also functions as a mirror. If your plate skews toward the heavy side, your body will reflect that.

Simple choices make it easier to bring your plate into balance.

PROTEINS   *75-150 calories*
legumes, eggs or egg whites, low- or nonfat dairy, seafood, meat

STARCHES   *100-200 calories*
whole grains, starchy vegetables (potatoes, sweet potatoes, corn, peas), tortillas, pasta, bread, cereal

VEGETABLES   *≥ 25 calories*
all non-starchy vegetables (carrots, cabbage, broccoli, etc.)

BEVERAGES   *≤ 10 calories*
water, tea, coffee, low-calorie beverages

SWEETENERS   *≤ 25 calories*
sugar, honey, molasses, maple syrup

FATS   *≤ 50 calories*
nuts, seeds, avocados, olives, coconut, whole-fat dairy, all vegetable oils and animal fats (lard, chicken fat)

SNACKS/FRUITS   *50-150 calories*
See page 41 for suggestions.

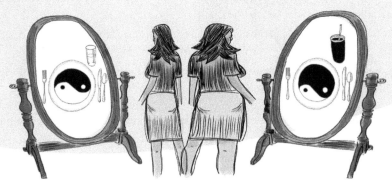

2   Food Sobriety takes a whole-body approach to weight loss.

Volume	Larger meals take up more room in your digestive system, causing a feeling of satiety that lasts.
Fiber	Fiber makes you feel full for longer. High-fiber foods also take longer to chew.
Digestion	The diet is high in whole foods, which causes the digestive tract to burn extra calories during digestion.
Eating Style	Eating slowly in a relaxed environment increases satiety.
Nutrient Balance	The mix of nutrients moderates blood sugar, which lowers cravings for calorie-dense foods.

These topics are covered in more detail in the coming chapters.

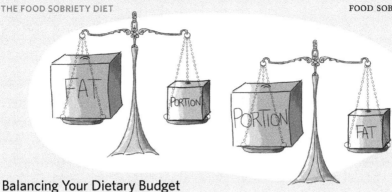

Balancing Your Dietary Budget

Having vegetables, protein, and at least some starch at meals is critical, so your big decision is between **fat** and **portion size**. I use a lower-fat, larger-portion diet as my default in this book but you can experiment with decreasing the portions and increasing the fat. Either strategy works well. The strategy that works better for you might be related to your genetics or might simply be a matter of taste.

What About Calories?

While individual needs vary, most people will experience significant weight loss eating between 1,200 and 1,800 calories per day. A rough guideline is to eat three meals a day that contain 300 to 500 calories each, and three snacks or fruits a day that vary from 50 to 150 calories per snack or fruit.

3   The Food Sobriety philosophy helps you put global health and nutrition shifts into context.

What caused the global obesity epidemic and how does that apply to you? In the last century, developments in food processing facilitated the inexpensive mass production of oil, flour, and sweeteners. Regardless of the specific foods you eat, keep these three categories to a minimum:

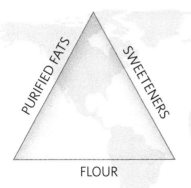

THE OBESITY TRIANGLE

Purified fats
All vegetable/seed oils, butter and margarine, and the foods made with them

Flour
Any foods made with flour (breads, pasta, crackers, noodles, bakery goods, etc.)

Sweeteners
All sweeteners (sugar, honey, molasses, etc.) and calorie-containing beverages, both processed (soda, fruit punch, energy drinks) and natural (juices, smoothies)

The Tortoise and the Hare

When I first starting working with overweight patients, I encouraged rapid overhauls of their diets and lifestyles. The patients who made radical changes saw stunning results, but tended to backslide over time. Patients who slowly adopted changes had the longest-lasting success, though their process took longer. My patients taught me that the most effective strategy is to make a series of small steps that gradually add up to a complete turnaround.

Behavioral physiologists believe that permanent changes in habit take between three and six months to cement. Once formed, good habits like loading up on veggies, checking labels, and eating mindfully (covered in Chapter 9) will become second nature.

The Tortoise: A Strategy for a Slow, Steady Transition to Food Sobriety

STAGE 1 1 TO 2 WEEKS

1 **Eat one Sober Plate meal a day** following the "how, when, and where" guidelines in Chapter 9. Pick the meal that you have the most time for. If your evenings are more relaxed than your mornings, do it in the evening. If you don't have a supportive environment at home, pick lunch (or whatever meal you often eat outside the home).

2 **Journal your diet** at least one day a week.

3 **Replace all beverages** with no- or low-calorie options (*< 10 calories per 8 ounces*).

STAGE 2 3 TO 6 WEEKS

4 **Every meal should have a representative from the three groups**. The proportions don't have to be precise, but the appearance of balance needs to begin.

5 **Make the switch** to low-fat cooking techniques and low-fat foods *(the leanest meat/fish and nonfat or low-fat dairy)* or choose higher-fat options and decrease your portion sizes.

6 **Eat at least half of your meals** following the "how, when, and where" guidelines.

STAGE 3 6 WEEKS TO PERMANENT

7 **The proportions now reflect the Sober Plate** at almost all meals.

8 **Eat almost all of your meals** following the "how, when, and where" guidelines.

9 **Replace desserts and sweet snacks** with low-calorie options.

The Food Sobriety Challenge: A 28-Day Dietary Overhaul

I recommend following the slow, steady path I just described, but no weight loss book is complete without a challenge. Returning to our political metaphor: can we simultaneously balance the budget, cut taxes, and expand government services? No—and likewise this dietary challenge comes with the mathematical constraint of limiting calories to between 1,200 and 1,800 per day (and a few other details—see below). Two versions of a weekly menu follow. Repeat either menu for a month and you will have completed the challenge.

The Menus

The **first menu**, featured in detail with photos, recipes, and calorie counts (pages 32-38), was inspired by the diet I ate in Nicaragua during my rapid weight loss in 2006. Because I add meat and a few North American health-food items it contains more variety, and more flavor, than what I ate in Nicaragua. Most of the meals feature a starch (corn, corn tortillas, or potatoes) and a legume (beans). This combination was the dietary foundation for tens of millions of indigenous people, including the Inca, Maya, Aztec, Pueblo, Cherokee, and Iroquois. The influence of this diet stretches from the Andes all the way to the Great Lakes, so I call it the Diet of the Americas.

The **second menu** (pages 39-40) is closer to a conventional North American diet. I don't stress specific serving sizes because everyone's needs are different and because following the Sober Plate proportions is the priority. Refer to the photos in the Diet of the Americas to get an idea of portion size.

Both menus stress simplicity. Cooking is a basic human skill, like being able to walk or talk. It shouldn't always require complicated recipes or more than a half-hour of work. I include a handful of favorite recipes in the Appendix. These "minimal effort, maximum nutrition" meals are simple enough that even the novice cook can be cooking up a storm within minutes.

 A Few Things to Keep in Mind

Most of my Sober Plate meals feature generous portions. This is possible because they are prepared using minimal fat. The daily menu also omits sweeteners and desserts. You may add either to your diet as long you keep calorie totals under control. Adding fat and sweets means smaller meal portions. (There are a few modest dessert options on page 40, and fats and sweets are discussed in detail in Chapter 8.)

Paying attention to your **plate size** is important. Most of the meals in the guide are on salad-size plates (nine-inch diameter).

The calorie totals don't include calorie-containing **condiments** like dressings and sauces. Pay attention to the amounts you use and adjust your total accordingly.

You can add up to three healthy **snacks** per day. See page 41.

DIET OF THE AMERICAS

BREAKFAST   359 calories

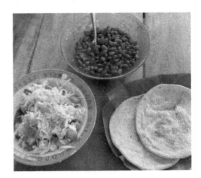

¼ head green cabbage
Your choice of veggies (*tomatoes, carrots, peppers, and onions are a good mix*)
1 T vinegar (*any kind you like*),
or a squeeze of lime juice
1 cup cooked beans
2 corn tortillas

Make a vegetable slaw: Shred the cabbage and dice the veggies. Mix together, toss with vinegar; let stand for a few minutes. Serve with beans and tortillas.

LUNCH   375 calories

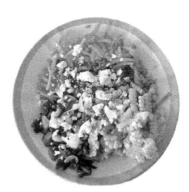

1 large carrot, shredded
1 ear corn, kernels removed, cooked
(or ¾ cup canned or frozen corn, cooked)
½ cup cooked beans
1-½ oz. crumbled soft cheese such as feta
½ orange
cilantro, salt, pepper

Mix veggies and beans in a bowl and add cheese. Squeeze the juice of the orange into the bowl and add cilantro, salt, and pepper to taste.

DINNER   364 calories

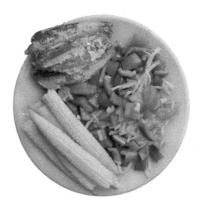

1 can sardines (4 oz.), packed in water
1 cup cooked corn (*see choices above*)
2 cups raw veggies (*carrot, tomatoes, bell pepper; about one each depending on size*)

Shred or grate carrot; dice tomatoes and peppers. Toss together and serve with corn and sardines. Add a low-calorie sauce or spices for flavoring.

The corn pictured is common in Latin America. Called "young corn," it is bigger than baby corn but much smaller than a mature ear of corn. Like baby corn, it is tender enough that you can eat the entire ear.

Monday   1,098 calories

DIET OF THE AMERICAS

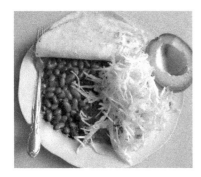

BREAKFAST   413 calories

1 cup cabbage slaw *(recipe previous page)*
¾ cup cooked beans
1 corn tortilla
½ avocado

Use salt, pepper, lime, herbs, and spices for flavor.

This breakfast goes lighter on the portions to make up for the high-fat, high-calorie avocado.

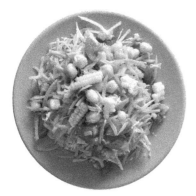

LUNCH   405 calories

1 large carrot, shredded or grated
¾ cup cooked garbanzo beans
1 cup cooked corn
¼ cup shredded, unsweetened coconut
1 medium tomato, chopped

Toss ingredients together. Add a low-calorie salad dressing or use vinegar with citrus juice, mint, salt, and pepper.

This is an example of a resistant starch salad. Resistant starches are covered in Chapter 5.

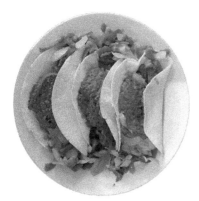

DINNER   423 calories

1 large green pepper	½ t paprika
1 large red pepper	½ T fat or oil
1 medium onion	½ cup fat-free refried beans
1 clove garlic, minced	2 T plain nonfat Greek yogurt
½ t red pepper flakes	3 T salsa
½ t dried oregano	3 corn tortillas

Preheat oven to 425°F. Dice vegetables and toss them with the seasonings and fat/oil. Spread them out on a nonstick baking pan and roast for 10-15 minutes. Lightly toast the tortillas. Heat up refried beans in a pan with just enough water to prevent them from sticking. Stuff each tortilla with 2-½ tablespoons of beans and another tablespoon or two of veggies. Line the plate with the leftover vegetables. Serve with salsa and plain Greek yogurt (in place of sour cream).

1 T whole-milk Greek yogurt = 2 T nonfat

Tuesday   1,241 calories

DIET OF THE AMERICAS

Breakfast   390 calories

2 cups fresh or frozen greens
(kale, spinach, or collard)
1 clove garlic, minced
2 eggs
2 slices toast *(approx. 50-60 calories per slice)*
½ cup pasta sauce, ¼ cup salsa

Steam greens with garlic, drain water. Poach eggs, toast bread, and serve with salsa over the greens and pasta sauce over the eggs and toast.

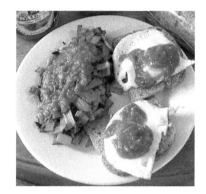

Lunch   457 calories

1 medium (6 oz.) potato
½ T oil or fat
1-½ cups veggie slaw
⅔ cup garbanzo beans

Preheat oven to 450°F. Cut potatoes into slices and place on a baking sheet brushed with the oil/fat. Bake until done (15-20 minutes).

Drizzle veggie slaw and beans with a low-calorie dressing (citrus-based works best). The potato slices go well with ketchup or tomato sauce — either 100% puréed tomatoes or a pasta sauce.

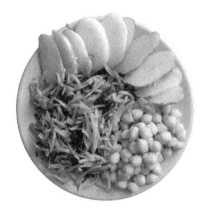

Dinner   304 calories

4 oz. white fish *(sole, flounder, cod, tilapia, haddock, and halibut are good choices)*
1 clove garlic, sliced
1 T fresh lime juice
onion powder, pepper (to taste)
parsley
¾ cup cooked brown rice
2 cups salad

Preheat oven to 450°F. Place fish on a sheet of parchment paper in a small baking dish. Sprinkle fish with lime juice, onion powder, sliced garlic, and pepper. Bake until fish flakes easily (about 4-6 minutes per ½-inch thickness). Sprinkle with parsley and serve with rice and salad.

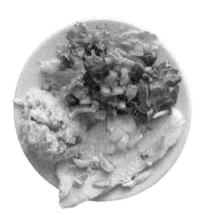

Wednesday   1,151 calories

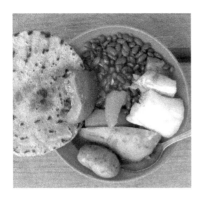

Breakfast   373 calories

¾ cup mixed steamed veggies (non-starchy)
¾ cup starchy veggies *(potatoes, yuca)*
¾ cup cooked beans
1 large corn tortilla

Good condiment choices are salsa and hot sauce
or crumbled cheese and nutritional yeast.

*Chayote, carrot, yuca, and mini-potato are
common in Nicaragua. Use any mix you like.*

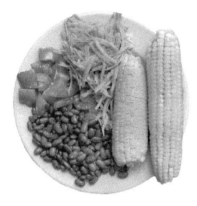

Lunch   405 calories

¾ cup cooked beans
1 cup shredded carrot
½ cup diced tomatoes
2 ears (or 1-½ cups) cooked corn

Add some flavor: Suggestions include 1 ounce of
chopped almonds, a light drizzle (½ tablespoon)
of olive oil, fresh citrus juice, salt, and pepper.

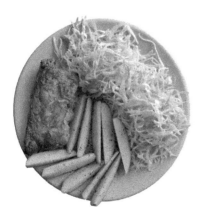

Dinner   409 calories

5 oz. chicken thigh, bone in, skin on
Low-calorie dressing or marinade
(citrus-based works well in this recipe)
1 medium (6 oz.) potato
½ T oil or fat
salt, pepper
2 cups cabbage salad

Marinate chicken for at least 30 minutes. Preheat
oven to 425°F. Remove chicken from marinade
and place on parchment in a small baking dish.
Bake until thoroughly cooked (at least 30 minutes or 160°F internal temperature). Serve with
boiled potato wedges or baked french fries (see
Wednesday lunch) and cabbage salad.

Thursday   1,187 calories

DIET OF THE AMERICAS

BREAKFAST   357 calories

1-½ cups green beans (fresh or frozen)
½ cup split peas
1 egg, poached or boiled
¾ cup of cooked corn

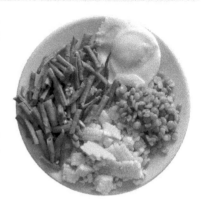

Steam green beans till soft. In a small pot, boil 1-½ cups of water, add the split peas, and return to boil. Reduce heat, partially cover pan, and simmer until slightly soft. Serve with the egg and steamed corn.

A mix of mustard and nutritional yeast makes a great flavoring for this breakfast. Split peas will cook more quickly if you soak them ahead of time

LUNCH   371 calories

2 cups mixed vegetables
4 oz. cooked chicken, cubed
¾ cup cooked rice
1 T soy sauce

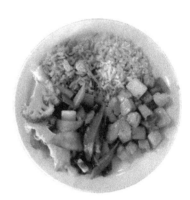

Steam the veggies in a shallow pan with enough water (about ½ cup) to keep the them from sticking. In the last minute or two add the soy sauce and chicken, and warm through. Serve with rice.

An easy shortcut is to buy a frozen vegetable stir-fry mix and precooked chicken strips.

DINNER   465 calories

⅔ cup cooked rice
1 cup cooked beans
½ cup sliced onions and tomatoes
½ T vinegar *(apple cider vinegar works well)*
½ cup vegetable or chicken broth
1 cup mixed vegetables
salt, pepper

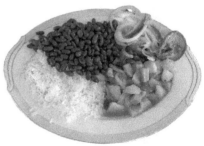

Toss tomatoes and onions with vinegar, salt, and pepper. In a small saucepan cook the mixed vegetables in the broth until slightly soft. Serve with rice and beans.

Friday   1,193 calories

DIET OF THE AMERICAS

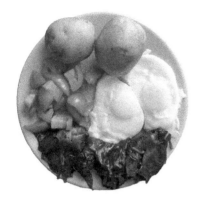

BREAKFAST   406 calories

2 eggs
2 small (4-5 oz.) potatoes
2 cups spinach (fresh or frozen)
1 medium tomato, diced

Poach or soft-boil eggs. Bake or boil potatoes till tender. Boil spinach 1-2 minutes. Serve with salsa or the flavoring of your choice.

A scoop of plain yogurt works well as a topping for the potatoes.

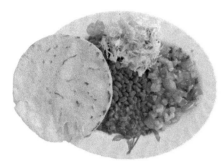

LUNCH   415 calories

2 medium tomatoes   1 large corn tortilla
1 small onion   1 cup cooked beans
1 small pepper   1 cup cabbage salad
¼ cup cilantro
1 lime, juiced

Make a quick *pico de gallo* to spice up your lunch: Dice tomatoes, onions, pepper, and cilantro. Place in a bowl and mix with the lime juice. Serve with the tortilla, beans, and cabbage salad.

DINNER   385 calories

5 oz. chicken thigh, bone in, skin on
low-calorie marinade *(citrus works well)*
1 cup cabbage salad
1 small tomato, diced
¼ avocado
1 large corn tortilla, rolled and cut into thirds

Marinate chicken for at least 30 minutes. Preheat oven to 425°F. Remove chicken from marinade, place on parchment in a small baking dish, and bake until cooked through (at least 30 minutes). Serve with the cabbage salad, tomatoes, avocado, and tortilla.

The higher fat from the skin on the chicken thigh and the avocado is balanced by smaller portions of carbohydrate (tortilla, 90 calories) and vegetables (very low-calorie cabbage salad)

Saturday   1,206 calories

DIET OF THE AMERICAS

BREAKFAST   420 calories

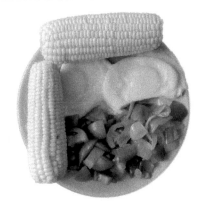

1 medium bell pepper, diced
1 small onion, diced
2 eggs, poached
2 ears (or 1-½ cups) cooked corn
2 small tomatoes, sliced

In a small pot with ½ cup of water or broth, simmer peppers and onions till soft. Serve with the
corn, eggs, and sliced tomatoes.

LUNCH   450 calories

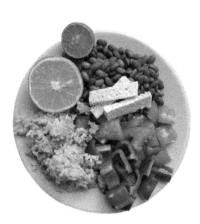

½ cup cooked beans
⅔ cup cooked brown rice
1 oz. cheese
2 medium tomatoes, diced
1 medium bell pepper, diced
½ small orange, ½ lime, juiced
salt, pepper

Serve as pictured. Use the fresh citrus juice, salt,
and pepper to flavor.

DINNER   424 calories

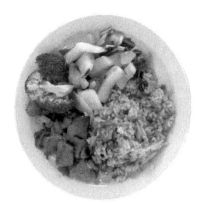

4 oz. lean beef medallions
low-calorie marinade/dressing
1 cup mixed ("Asian-style") stir-fry vegetables
½ cup broccoli
1 cup rice pilaf (store-bought mix)

Marinate beef for at least 30 minutes. Cook pilaf
mix with bouillon or a mix of dried or fresh herbs.
Grill beef (use a George Foreman or other nonstick electric grill) until done, at least 5-10 minutes,
depending on the thickness of the beef. In a small,
uncovered pot with about ½ cup of water or broth,
simmer veggies until tender.

Sunday   1,294 calories

CONVENTIONAL DIET

BREAKFASTS

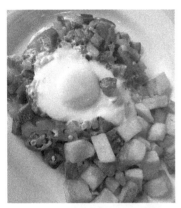

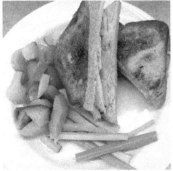

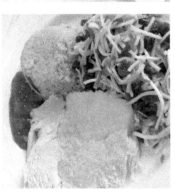

MON	Hard-boiled egg sandwich: 2 eggs, 2 pieces of toast, steamed greens, tomato, mustard; side dish of sauerkraut
TUE	2 whole-grain pancakes (4-inch), egg white scramble with tomatoes and peppers
WED	2-egg omelet filled with vegetable mix, small pieces of toast
THU	Beans, 1 poached egg, baked potato, steamed spinach
FRI	Veggie burger on toast with tomato, onion, lettuce, and a side salad
SAT	Roasted veggies with a poached egg and baked hash browns
SUN	2 poached eggs, brown rice, steamed broccoli, and cauliflower with garlic and onions

LUNCHES

MON	Large split pea soup, baked sweet potato
TUE	Shrimp ceviche,* crackers
WED	Turkey sandwich, steamed vegetables
THU	Steamed spinach, medium bowl of lentil soup, rice
FRI	Small chicken burrito, sugar snap peas
SAT	Bowl of chili, steamed veggies
SUN	Extra-lean turkey burger* on a whole-wheat bun, with salad and a cup of sauerkraut

Recipes for items marked with * can be found in the Appendix, pp. 193-206.

DINNERS

MON	Roast turkey, quinoa, mixed root veggie slaw with raisins
TUE	Roasted mushrooms and cauliflower, bowl of chili, baked potato
WED	Pork chop with applesauce, baked french fries, salad
THU	Grilled chicken, small boiled potatoes, mixed peas and carrots
FRI	Healthy and easy pizza,* salad
SAT	Grilled shrimp, baked sweet potato, carrot salad*
SUN	Veggie burger* on a multigrain bun, squash soup*

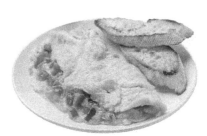

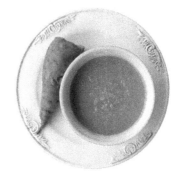

DESSERTS

Fruit salad

Frozen yogurt

Frozen fruit popsicles

Frozen banana ice cream*

Low-calorie (or agar) jello*

Baked apples with cinnamon

Chocolate-covered strawberries

Chocolate-covered frozen bananas

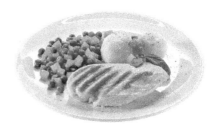

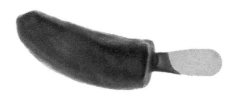

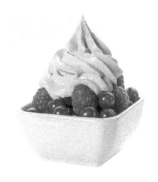

Snacks and Fruit

You probably noticed that the daily menus don't mention snacks or fruit. Because those menus average only about 1,200 calories, there is room for you to add a few hundred calories a day.

Pair a light (veggies) with a heavy (starch and/or protein); add a condiment if you like.

Light	Heavy		
VEGGIES	STARCH	PROTEIN	CONDIMENT
Carrot sticks	Baked tortilla chips	Low-fat hummus*	Lime
Celery	Brown rice cakes	Black bean dip*	Mustard
Steamed broccoli	Whole wheat pretzels	Low-fat cream cheese	Puréed tomatoes
Tomato slices	Toast	Yogurt dressing	Salsa
Sugar snap peas	Baked french fries	Plain yogurt	Peanut butter-ginger sauce
Jicama	Sweet potato fries	Low-fat cheese	
Fresh fruit	Corn tortillas		*(More ideas on p. 42)*

Shoot for snacks that are between 50 and 150 calories. Examples:

Carrot sticks with hummus	Sugar snap peas with yogurt dressing
Celery with black bean dip	Jicama with lime
Baked tortilla chips with salsa	Plain yogurt with fresh fruit
Steamed broccoli with peanut butter-ginger sauce	Whole wheat pretzels with mustard
Baked french fries or sweet potatoes with puréed tomatoes (or ketchup)	Toast with sliced tomatoes and low-fat cheese
Brown rice cakes with low-fat cream cheese and tomato slices	Mini-pizza: toasted tortilla with tomato sauce and low-fat cheese

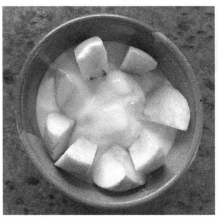 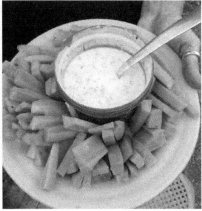

Flavorings/Condiments

The Food Sobriety menus keep the recipes simple and the flavoring options to a minimum. The simplicity is for ease of meal preparation and to encourage experimentation; use these suggestions to tailor the diets to suit your taste.

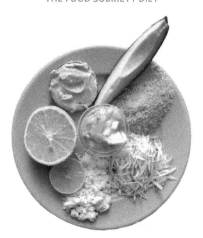

When you prepare foods with a minimum of time, effort, and fat, it helps to have low-calorie flavors ready to add at the table.

Experiment with condiments:

Salsa	From mild to hot, fresh or pre-packaged
Nutritional yeast	Tastes like parmesan cheese and is packed with protein
Horseradish	Clears the sinuses and adds a kick to sauces and dressings
Herbs, spices	Fresh and dried, pre-made mixes (like Mrs. Dash), and classics like onion powder, garlic powder, basil, and oregano
Tomato sauce	The best is 100% puréed tomatoes. If you prefer pasta sauce, look for those made without oil and sweeteners.
Mustard	Whole-grain mustard is best but Dijon is also quite tasty
Barbeque sauce	Look for one low in sugar and fat
Vinegar	There are so many wonderful kinds. Experiment!
Fresh citrus	Lemons, limes, and oranges
Dressings and marinades	Look for dressings with no or minimal oil; yogurt- or fruit based is best. Most dressings work well as marinades, too. Try a couple of teaspoons of alcohol in a marinade to add flavor (rum and whiskey work well).
Sauces	Many sauces used in Asian cuisine work well. Try soy and ginger-soy, teriyaki, Vietnamese fish sauce, and Thai flavors. Don't forget your favorite hot sauce!

Condiment plate, clockwise from top left: mustard, avocado, nutritional yeast, shredded coconut, crumbled feta, lime, orange; center: onions in vinegar

Quick Guide and Cooking Tips

When your meal calls for **beans**, try

Method/Type	How-to	Good choices
Soaked, cooked	See Appendix	Pinto, black, Great Northern, navy, garbanzo
Canned, whole	Rinse and heat	Any kind with little or no added oil
Sprouted	See Appendix	Mung, garbanzo, azuki

When you're cooking **eggs**, try

Method	How-to
Soft/hard boiled	Boil for 5 to 10 minutes depending on how much you like the yolk cooked
Over easy	Use a nonstick pan or use cooking spray instead of oil
Poached	Crack into a pan containing 1 inch of boiling water, cover, cook for 5-7 minutes

When you're cooking **corn**, try

Type	How-to
Fresh, on the cob	Microwave 4-6 minutes on high; boil 5 minutes until tender; grill; roast
Frozen, bagged	Follow directions on package
Canned or jarred	Rinse and warm up or eat as is for cold dishes

Avoid canned corn with added sugar, oil, or added flavoring. A squeeze of lime tastes great on corn.

Try **roasting** your vegetables

How-to	Veggies	Time
Toss in a bowl with a little olive oil (less than ½ T of olive oil per cup of vegetables) and turn out onto a rimmed baking sheet lined with a silicone mat or parchment paper. (No liner is needed with a nonstick baking sheet.) Roast at 425°F on the top rack of the oven until golden brown; season to taste.	Root vegetables and tubers (potatoes, carrots, beets)	30-45 minutes if whole, less if cut into pieces
	Eggplant, squash, cauliflower, broccoli, brussels sprouts, bell peppers, tomatoes	15-20 minutes
	Green beans, asparagus	10-20 minutes

- *Toast tortillas* before serving. A little crispiness makes even the dullest store-bought tortilla come alive. Look for tortillas between 40 and 50 calories each.
- Make lots of *veggie slaw or cabbage salad* at the beginning of the week — it'll stay fresh for at least 4 to 5 days and you can eat it with many meals. The same goes for legumes and grains.
- A good rule of thumb for *baking fish* is 4-6 minutes at 425°F for every half-inch thickness of the fillet (e.g., a 1-inch thick fillet would cook in about 8-12 minutes).

  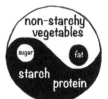 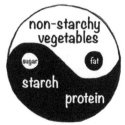

As your sugar intake and fat intake decrease, your portion size can increase.

If you think cooking is inconvenient...

In many parts of the world, people have to cut firewood and haul it home in order to cook. In rural areas of the developing world, including Nicaragua, burning wood for cooking creates two problems: deforestation and eye and lung damage from daily smoke exposure.

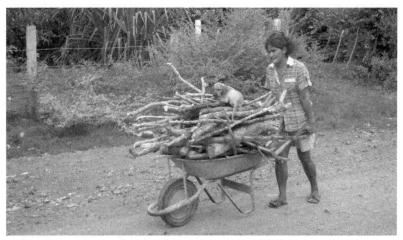

In Las Palmas, a woman transports a few days worth of firewood (and a hitchhiker).

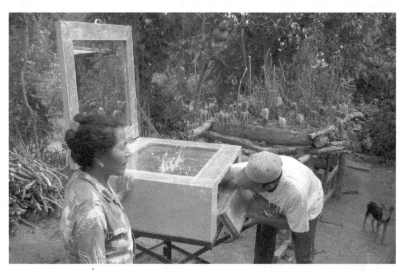

This couple in Totogalpa uses a solar oven provided by Grupo Fenix, a Nicaraguan nonprofit that focuses on sustainable development. In sunny, warm climates solar ovens cook meals in a few hours. Solar ovens are also healthier, as they promote baking rather than frying.

CHAPTER 4

Calorie Conundrums
How Diets Do and Don't Fill You

TO LOSE WEIGHT WE SHOULD FOLLOW THE THREE DIETARY RULES: eat fewer calories than we burn, meet our nutritional needs, and follow a diet that satisfies us. That's it, right? Yes, but that last point is the ultimate example of the devil in the details. When we eat fewer calories than we burn, our body tends to compensate by increasing our appetite. When we can't satisfy our appetite, we eventually succumb to unhealthy choices and the weight returns. This chapter explores the relationships between calories, digestion, and satiety in order to demonstrate how to maximize every opportunity to feel full.

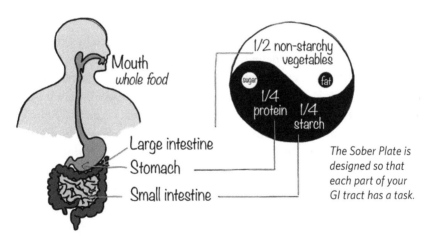

The Sober Plate is designed so that each part of your GI tract has a task.

The Gastrointestinal Tract Full Employment Program

The digestive tract is a *disassembly* line. As we eat, segments of our meal are continually rolling down the tract while digestive work specific to each organ's function frees up nutrients for absorption. The steady pace and evenly divided workload created by a balanced meal contribute to long-lasting satiety. Additionally, when the GI tract is fully occupied more calories are burned during the digestive process.

With every balanced **Sober Plate meal**:

1. Your **mouth** is engaged by food that requires chewing: whole foods that have not been softened, ground up, or otherwise processed.

2. Your **stomach** is engaged by protein. Protein's complex structure is unwound by stomach acid into digestible fragments.

3. Your **small intestine** is engaged by starch. The unrefined starches emphasized in the Food Sobriety diet are mostly complex carbohydrates, whose long polysaccharide chains take time to break down.

4. Your **large intestine** processes the fiber and reabsorbs water. Vegetables are mostly composed of fiber and water, ensuring a busy large intestine.

There Are Calories — and Then There Are Calories

Let's tackle that second rule of weight loss. Now that our plate is balanced, all we need to do is eat fewer calories than we burn, right? Yes, but again, the details matter. Consider these two questions, both critical for weight loss:

1. How full does a food make you feel?

2. How many calories are burned in the digestion process?

Calories are fuel, like gasoline or electricity; they are measured by the energy they provide. The textbook definition of a **calorie** is the amount of energy needed to raise the temperature of one gram of water by one degree Celsius. Another way to think of calories is that they are the unit we use to measure a food's capacity to fuel the activities of life. However, a calorie's capacity to make us feel full varies greatly, and our technique for measuring calories is not capable of accounting for this. The number of calories burned in the process of digestion is known as the **thermic effect** of food. Calorie numbers are calculated using a machine called a bomb calorimeter, which accurately measures the energy contained in food by burning it under controlled conditions. The calorimeter, however, is not a replica of the human digestive tract, and it fails to address our two critical questions.

Throughout the following chapters I will refer to those two factors to explain how you can make choices that burn the most calories (increase the thermic effect) and maximize fullness. In the future, perhaps our food labels will

 You'll see this graphic and the term MPC (minutes per calorie) when I estimate the amount of time the calories in a given food will make us feel full. MPC is the "satiety mileage" we get out of calories, a way to combine the concepts of thermic effect and satiety.

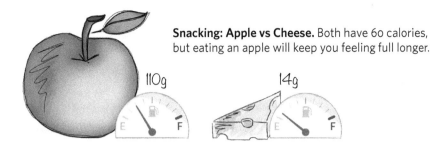

Snacking: Apple vs Cheese. Both have 60 calories, but eating an apple will keep you feeling full longer.

110g

14g

account for the difference between the way calories are measured and the effect they have. Until then, we need to be mindful that a calorie is a measure of total energy contained, not a measure of net energy (calories minus the thermic effect) or **satiety**.

Innovation Doesn't Always Mean Improvement

It helps to look at the bigger picture. We always face the same dilemma: how to fuel our economies and ourselves. Fuel sources, whether for machines or humans, tend to follow a long-term trend of becoming continually more concentrated and cheaper. Concentrated fuels yield more energy and are easier to control, if not monopolize entirely. Until recently there has been little interest in less-concentrated fuel sources. In fact, there is no common form of food processing that decreases calorie density or increases the thermic effect.

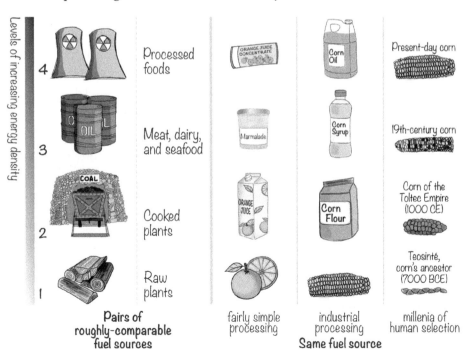

Increasing fuel densities are matched by increasing consolidation of the business network involved in the production, transport, distribution, and sale of food and fuel. This trend has increased the distance between the consumer and the production and management of our fuels. As people seek a closer, more secure connection to fuels, far-flung oil fields are slowly yielding to rooftop solar panels and domestic wind farms. Likewise, people are comparing the merits of industrial food with those of locally grown, less processed, and thus, less energy-dense food. The realization that not every innovation, not every efficiency, is a qualitative upgrade is occasionally reflected in popular culture. Aficionados of authenticity turn off their digital devices and explore the warm crackle of vinyl records and the creased pages of a well-thumbed book.

From Leaves to Steak

The trend to more concentrated energy sources stretches so far back that it is a defining trait of our evolution. Our primate ancestors had long digestive tracts because their diet, raw plants, required a great deal of digestive labor. They also spent most of the day gathering food and chewing because raw plants have both minimal caloric density and a high thermic effect. In other words, it takes a big pile of leaves to keep meat on the bones. In *Catching Fire: How Cooking Made Us Human*, biological anthropologist and Harvard professor Richard Wrangham fills in the details: "Carnivores, such as dogs and wolves, have smaller intestines than plant eaters, such as horses, cows, or antelopes [...]. In species that are adapted to eating more easily-digested foods, such as sugar-rich fruits compared to fibrous leaves, guts are also relatively small: fruit-eating chimpanzees or spider monkeys have smaller guts than the leaf-eating gorillas or howler monkeys. Those reduced guts use less total energy than larger guts."

Our evolution is characterized by the struggle to obtain enough calories. Any innovation that made it easier to consume more calories or break them down more rapidly (decrease the thermic effect) was adopted. The most effective method to increase caloric density is to process food. The first form of processing was an extension of our teeth—smashing up foods with small wooden and stone tools. With less chewing there was a gradual decrease in the size of our jaws and facial muscles.

The next step was cooking, which originated with our ancestor *Homo habilis* well over a million years ago. Cooking acts like an external organ of our body, a "pre-stomach." Cooked food lowers the thermic effect because it requires less chewing, stomach acid, intestinal churning, and digestive enzymes. Anthropologists like Wrangham believe that as cooking incrementally increased, our digestive tracts shortened and the resulting energy surplus was used to grow our brains. With more powerful brains we innovated ways to prepare food to maximize caloric density. We even discovered additional calorie sources. Because of its high calorie density, the most important new source was meat, which involved the novel, complex, and cooperative activity of hunting and using weapons.

What does this detour into evolutionary biology have to do with weight? If the farther we get from eating raw, whole food—eating increasingly more processed foods—decreases the calories we burn in digestion and helps us gain weight, then the opposite is also true. *Eating less-processed foods burns more calories (increases the thermic effect) and reduces weight.* I'm not suggesting that we should all return to chewing on leaves, but we should account for the degree of processing our food undergoes and how that affects weight.

Nuclear Energy — Flour and Isolated Fats

We've all heard enough from finger-wagging health experts about sweeteners and white flour to know that these are trouble. What has escaped scrutiny is that all refined carbohydrates and isolated fats do the same thing: promote weight gain. Don't be fooled by boutique flours (gluten-free, barley, coconut, almond, rice, etc.). These might be healthy choices when weight is not an issue, but, like cooking, grinding foods into tiny particles of flour is another method of pre-digesting. Flour and products made with flour are digested quickly, yielding a low MPC.

Likewise, concentrated fats isolate the fat from dairy, nuts, seeds, and grains and leave the fiber, protein, water, and complex carbohydrates behind. The fewer pure fats such as butter, margarine, and oil your diet has, the easier your weight loss will be. As above, although the source of your fat has implications for general health, where weight loss is concerned both cheap margarine and organic, extra-virgin olive oil are best used sparingly.

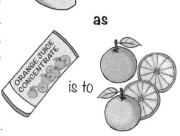

Fats and sweeteners are discussed in more detail in **Chapter 8**.

Baby Food for Adults, Hospital Food for the Healthy

One day a few summers ago, I was conducting a grocery store tour for a group of clients. As I walked through the aisles pointing out useful foods and shortcuts to make convenient meals, a 45-year-old social worker named Kim stopped me. I had just dismissed several shelves of energy bars with a quick wave, stating, "These pack on the pounds, you eat them in minutes, and they don't keep you full. They're calorie grenades." Kim tugged on my arm, pleading, "Dan, I *love* bars, please just tell me the best one." I responded, "Kim, I can't. They're sliced-up, pre-digested food elements mashed together with sticky sweeteners. Think of this as a baby food aisle for adults." Undeterred, Kim continued protesting, "I just want something I can eat really quick. I don't have any time; I need something I don't have to think about."

Calorie Grenades

If you cut corners to quickly put something in your stomach, you won't feel full for long. Energy bars, trail mix, granola, protein shakes, smoothies, and sports drinks were all developed to meet the needs of athletes who were burning large quantities of calories and found it difficult to consume enough calories in a regular diet to keep the pounds on. Athletes benefit from low-MPC, calorie-dense snacks that are digested quickly and don't make them feel full, allowing a quick return to training. (When we digest a meal, some of our blood flow is redirected to our intestinal tract. The quicker a food is digested, the quicker our blood flow can be redirected to our muscles. Incidentally, this is why you shouldn't exercise vigorously right after you've eaten—both your digestion and your muscular function will be compromised.)

By processing food into powders, shakes, and bars, manufacturers are essentially **pre-digesting** it for us. Processing breaks down the structure, the low-calorie elements (vegetable matter), and removes the water. The result is food that takes minimal digestive effort, even minimal chewing. The allure of these snack foods for those who aren't athletes is that you can quickly munch (or slurp) them while multitasking. *I only recommend these foods to athletes, people recovering from illness or surgery, underweight pregnant women, and others at risk of under-consuming calories.*

The manufacturers of shortcut foods associate their products with sports and intense exercise, even though most consumers are not exercising nearly enough to benefit from using these products. The makers of "Ensure" and other meal-replacement drinks similarly exploit the medical origins of their products. These products were developed for hospitalized patients whose medical conditions required high calorie intake to promote recovery. Patients often couldn't meet these calorie and nutrient goals with solid food because of a lack of appetite or compromised digestion. For this same reason hospitals were the most enthusiastic adopters of the earliest blender prototypes in the 1930s and '40s. Then, as now, blended drinks were used primarily as a way to increase calorie intake and to provide a respite for the digestive tract.

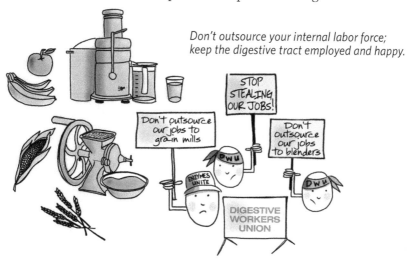

Don't outsource your internal labor force; keep the digestive tract employed and happy.

What About Beverages?

While processed foods have a lower thermic value than whole foods, liquefied foods have an even lower value. If you use a juicer or blender to prepare a drink, the blades of the blender or the whirring motor of the extractor is doing the job of your mouth and GI tract, reducing the MPC. Again, it is the work of digestion that both burns calories and creates a sense of fullness. Don't outsource your internal labor force; keep your digestive tract employed and happy.

Oranges to Oranges

A 12-ounce glass of orange juice and three medium-large oranges both contain about 160 calories.

How long does it take you to drink a 12-ounce glass of orange juice — five or 10 minutes? Do you feel full after drinking it?

How long does it take you to peel, chew and eat three oranges? (It will take you at least twice as long and you will feel full for *much* longer.)

- **Avoid** juices, smoothies, yogurt drinks, sodas, energy drinks, and vitamin-enhanced waters. Stick to drinks with very few calories (10 calories or fewer per eight ounces) or no calories: herbal teas, carbonated water, mineral water, and naturally flavored waters.

- If you're transitioning from a diet full of strongly flavored beverages, **give your taste buds some time to adjust.** Begin by diluting juice and other sweet beverages with water, adjusting the ratio by a slight amount daily. I have had many patients try this, and by the end of a month they are using only small amounts of juice to "paint" the water.

Does Soup Count as a Beverage?

No. Most soups are served hot, need some chewing (unless they're puréed or only broth), and are eaten with a spoon. These factors mean that a 16-ounce portion of soup takes a while to eat, whereas a 16-ounce beverage goes down quickly. The composition of soup is also different; the calories in soup don't come solely from simple carbohydrates, as they usually do in beverages. Soups generally contain a mix of protein, carbohydrate, and fat. When buying pre-made soups, look for soups with fewer than 120 calories per cup.

Hydration

The internal drives for thirst and hunger are intertwined: thirst stimulates the appetite, so it is common to think that you are hungry when you are actually dehydrated. However, when I tell my patients about the importance of hydration, their response is "I don't like the taste of water."

How could we lose our taste for water? Our species drank water, and *only* water, for hundreds of thousands of years. Three-quarters of our body weight is water, and three-quarters of the earth is water. All animals—indeed almost every living organism—consume water. We are the blue planet. If the Earth had a flag there would be water on it. If we had a sports team, it would be called The Flood. If we had a mascot it would be…well, you get the point.

DIY Low-Calorie Drinks

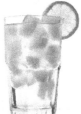

1. Fill a pitcher with water.

2. Add any of the following: lemons, limes, parsley, basil, strawberries — even cucumber slices.

3. Add a touch of non-caloric sweetener,* refrigerate, and you have your own low-cost, fancy drink.

* Discussed in Chapter 8

Water's Fall and the Three "C's"

Contamination

Our water supplies include many elements that alter water's taste. This is true even in a place like Nicaragua, where both the nat ural (volcanic soil) and the man-made (chemicals from agricultur-al run-off and factory waste) influence water's taste.

Competition

Water must compete with a wide variety of beverages. The complex tastes, textures, colors, and fragrances make water seem lackluster by comparison.

Containers

Water picks up the taste of plastic and metal. Drink filtered water and drink out of glass or ceramic containers.

Everything is harder when you're short on water.

Rather than having a specific daily goal for water consumption:

- Always **carry zero-calorie beverages** with you. Keep one in your car, office, purse, or backpack. Drink frequently—take sips even when you're not thirsty.

- Make it a habit to **keep hydrated**, and be conscious of the symptoms of dehy-dration: headaches, dry skin, dry mouth, fatigue, dizziness, frequent urinary tract infections, and muscle cramps. If you wear jewelry or a sports monitor, check how tight it feels in the morning and whether it feels looser later in the day. If it is, you are dehydrated. Your skin is one of the first places from which your body will lose water (and volume).

- **Monitor the color of your urine.** If it's often dark and concentrated you're not drinking enough water. If it's a light color or clear, you're fine. *Note:* Most vitamin supplements will give your urine a fluo-rescent yellow color. This has nothing to do with hydration status. It is excess ri-boflavin (vitamin B2), and the color will disappear in a few hours.

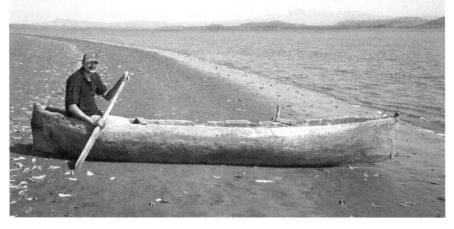

CHAPTER 5

Starches

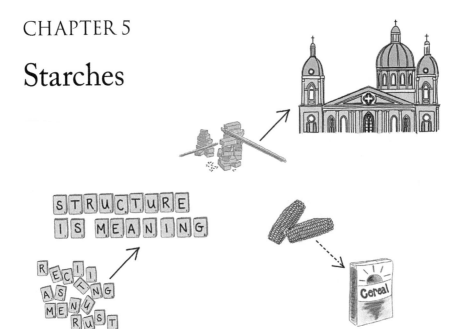

WEIGHT LOSS EXPERTS HAVE DEBATED THE ROLE OF STARCHES for decades. Starches have been both demonized as pound-packing villains and hailed as energy-boosting heroes. **Starches,** by definition, are types of carbohydrate made from different arrangements of glucose. They offer easily digestible energy and provide immediate satisfaction. A diet that has too much starch can cause weight gain because starch doesn't satiate long-term hunger and it causes insulin production. (**Insulin** is a hormone that, when produced in excess, signals your body to store more fat.)

If you're using the Sober Plate method, you'll find that a quarter-plate of starch (about 100-200 calories) will support your energy levels and, if you choose your starches well, will also aid in weight loss.

Most people are familiar with the term "carbs" as applied to diets. Here I'm referring to **starchy carbs**. Fruits, vegetables, and sweeteners are covered in Chapters 6 and 8.

Before I discuss the spectrum of starches, let's take a look at the anti-starch philosophies.

Low-Carbohydrate Diets

Diets that cut out most carbohydrates (like Atkins and Paleo) will cause rapid weight loss, but there are drawbacks:

1   Most people struggle to maintain the diet long term. When they give up, the weight returns quickly. One reason for the quick rebound on weight is that carbohydrates stored in our bodies are in a form called **glycogen**. Every gram of glycogen is stored with three to four grams of water, so when we use up our stores of it we can drop a dozen or so pounds of water weight. This loss accounts for the "miracle" effect during the first weeks of dieting. The water weight returns when you resume eating carbs.

2   The metabolic state of **ketosis** accompanies diets that consistently drop below 100 grams of carbohydrate per day. Signs of ketosis include bad breath, gas, low energy, weakness, and nausea. In some studies, long-term ketosis has been linked to damage to the liver, kidneys, and bones.

3   The bulk of the diet shifts to either fat or protein, both of which in excess are dangerous. High amounts of fat slow blood circulation, contribute to arterial blockages, burden the liver, and endanger cardiovascular health. High protein carries risks for kidney and bone health (see Chapter 7).

4   Unpleasant side effects are common: fatigue, low energy, digestive disturbances, and decrease in brain function ("brain fog").

Some years ago the Atkins diet was surpassed in popularity by the Paleo diet. The Paleo diet allows fruits and prohibits dairy, and Atkins has the opposite policy. Aside from that the diets are similar. The Paleo ethos is to avoid all foods that were (supposedly) not everyday staples prior to the advent of agriculture—the end of the Paleolithic period, approximately ten thousand years ago. Typical Paleo diets eliminate dairy, wheat, rice, oats, barley, rye, millet, corn, legumes, and starchy tubers like potatoes and cassava. Whether or not modern Paleo enthusiasts are actually eating a diet that resembles that of our ancestors, and whether it is wise to mimic the diet of people with half our current life expectancy, are subjects that stir much debate. I will leave that hornet's nest unpoked and instead focus on the positives and negatives.

Anthropologists believe that legumes and grains *were* common foods in the Paleolithic era, but were gathered from the wild rather than farmed.

Positives

1   Those who are sensitive to dairy and grains have improved digestion, develop strengthened immunity, and see a decrease in allergic responses.

2   Most adherents lose weight for as long as they can stick with the diet.

3   Like Atkins, Paleo eliminates a host of weight-promoting foods, among them most sweeteners, alcohol, cheese, pizza, and pastries.

Negatives

1   It is unnecessary for people who tolerate grains and/or dairy well.

2   The restrictions are immensely challenging to maintain.

3   While some thrive on the diet, others have the same complaints that can accompany Atkins: fatigue, digestive disturbances, and brain fog.

4   If carbohydrate intake falls far enough, ketosis begins.

5   Your animal-loving, environmentalist friends will harass you endlessly.

The Paleo diet owes some of its success to the attractive notion that if you follow the diet you will become the muscled Paleo person. The issue with taking a diet from an era or people and recreating it in another time and place is that the world has changed. We don't live the active lives of Paleolithic people. We face different stresses and challenges, and our food supply is radically different. For example, modern animals, on average, have far more fat than in the Paleolithic era, and our fruits are much sweeter and larger. As mentioned in Chapter 4, even our digestive tracts have evolved. While I don't promote (or denigrate) Paleo diets, I can recommend some "Paleo-esque" experimentation. Try a week or two without grains, dairy, or **gluten** (the protein found in wheat, barley, and rye). For some people these foods cause inflammation, and their elimination will result in a host of benefits, including weight loss. For others there will be no difference.

Raising animals for meat, even when done in the most environmentally sensitive manner, uses far more resources than growing other foods (vegetables, grains, legumes, and fruit).

Starches: The Ugly, the Good, and the Best

The Ugly: No Pain, All Gain

If there is one thing that both "meatetarians" and dietitians agree on it is to avoid **refined carbohydrates**. As I mentioned in Chapter 3, minimize your consumption of any kind of flour: pastries (muffins, croissants, biscuits, scones, cinnamon buns, etc.), breads, pasta, white rice, bagels, most crackers, and chips. It doesn't matter if the flour was made from organic coconut and blessed by a didgeridoo-jamming shaman. Flour, like oil, is an innovation produced by calorie-deprived populaces who sought to maximize caloric density.

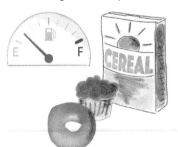

MPC = minutes per calorie; how long the calories in a given food will make us feel full

Breakfast cereals fall into the ugly category. Their grains have been cooked, compressed, sweetened, colored, glued together, and pressed into shapes. By the time cereal reaches your bowl the original grains have morphed into predigested food pellets that will pass rapidly through your intestinal tract. Cereals have a low thermic effect and a low MPC. Those that purport to be low calorie have often been subjected to one more processing step: inflating the grain with air. Puffed-up grains are low calorie, but the puffs offer minimal satisfaction because they are digested rapidly.

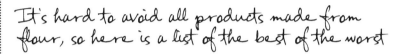

It's hard to avoid all products made from flour, so here is a list of the best of the worst

1   Multigrain pancakes (Kashi and Fiber One make some good mixes)

2   Whole-grain noodles (buckwheat, soba, whole wheat)

3   Whole wheat pasta

4   Corn or whole-wheat tortillas

5   Some crackers and breads. **Crackers**, like pasta and bread, are made primarily from flour. Although flour-based products are concentrated and highly processed, you can find a handful of fairly high-fiber, low-calorie crackers. Wasa and Ak-Mak are two of the best examples. **Whole-grain breads** should have at least three grams of fiber and between 50 and 80 calories per slice. A **better option** for breads are those made from sprouted grains. Try Ezekiel, Alvarado Street, and Trader Joe's store brand. These breads are both filling and quite low in calories. The only caveat with sprouted breads is that they don't taste like much right out of the package. Toast them to bring out their nutty, crunchy, sweet flavor.

6   One of the best **cereal alternatives** is steel-cut oats, also called "Irish oats." (They're discussed in the next section.) These are not rolled oats but little "pebbles" that look like genuine horse food. They usually take 45 minutes to cook, but if you soak them in water overnight they will cook in five to 10 minutes the following morning. They taste great hot, but they're versatile: try mixing cold leftover oats into yogurt and adding a touch of stevia, cinnamon, and vanilla extract. The result is a delicious tapioca-like dish.

7   If you crave a more traditional cold breakfast cereal, look for one with more than five grams of fiber and fewer than 120 calories per cup (serving sizes on the label will vary).

For more on stevia and other alternative sweeteners, see **Chapter 8**.

The Good: Resistant Starch, Moderate MPC

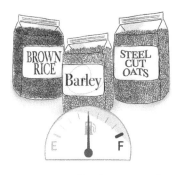

In this category are whole grains. Most of these good starches contain **resistant starch**, a type of starch that behaves more like fiber when digested. Unlike other starches, it passes largely intact through the small intestine. In the large intestine it becomes food for the resident beneficial bacteria. Resistant starch yields only two to three calories per gram, unlike other carbohydrates, which yield four calories per gram. The best sources of resistant starch are intact grains and legumes—not processed, cut, diced, or flattened. Resistant starch is destroyed in the milling process.

Another way to increase resistant starch in the diet is to eat starches that have been cooled after cooking. The temperature changes convert some regular starch into resistant starch. This works for a variety of foods. Cold potatoes, rice, pasta, and toast have more resistant starch than their warm versions. The news gets even better: since resistant starch is not affected by reheating, being lazy actually pays off. Leftovers—whether reheated or eaten cold—can help with weight loss.

It's a good idea to soak grains prior to cooking. Soaking increases digestibility, reduces cooking time, reduces **lectins** (a protein type that can cause digestive problems), and eliminates **phytic acid** (a nutrient that inhibits mineral absorption). Soaking time can vary from 20 minutes to a few hours, depending on which grain you're cooking.

All **whole grains** (but *not* "whole-grain products") are good choices, including barley, brown rice, bulgur wheat, wild rice, steel-cut oats, amaranth, buckwheat, and quinoa.

> **Experiment:** Compare how full you feel after eating a 150-calorie serving of steel-cut oats (one cup cooked) and after eating a 150-calorie serving of instant oats (¾ cup cooked; because the oat pieces are smaller, they pack down more). The smaller surface area and more intact grains of the steel-cut oats mean more resistant starch, more chewing, and more time and calories spent in your gastrointestinal tract, all of which make you feel full longer.

Legumes contain carbohydrate but are high in protein. I cover them in **Chapter 7**.

Chapter 3 has several dishes with high resistant starch, and you can find recipes in the **Appendix**.

The Best: High-MPC Foods

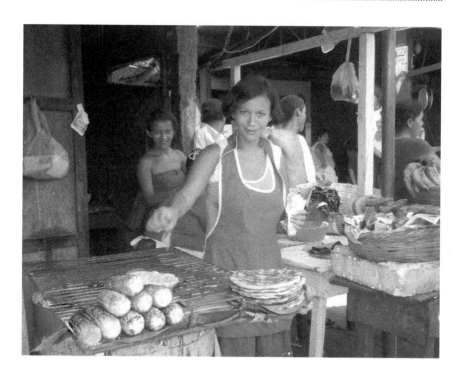

The best starches for weight loss include several foods that are traditionally categorized as vegetables. Though they may have been demonized in the past, these starches are only problematic on the Sober Plate if you count them as vegetables. For example, you are doubling up on starches if you eat both pasta and potatoes or corn and rice in the same meal.

With that caveat in mind, these fiber- and water-filled, stomach-satisfying starches are the **most potent weight loss starches available**: potatoes, pumpkin, corn, beets, sweet potatoes, parsnips, and squash.

Corn on the cob or güirila? Yessica sells carbohydrates on both ends of the spectrum. An ear of corn is a whole food and offers stomach-filling volume with minimal calories — an ideal starch for weight loss. The *güirila* is a large tortilla made from sweet young corn mixed with cheese and sugar, fried, and served with more cheese and sour cream. It is much higher in calorie density. The güirila is a refined food, best reserved as an occasional indulgence for those who are slim or highly active. (*Leon*)

CHAPTER 6

Vegetables

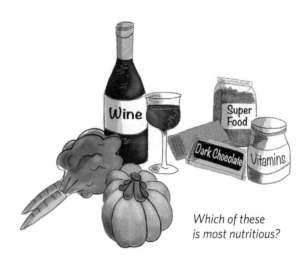

Which of these
is most nutritious?

THERE IS NOTHING MORE SOBER IN THE KINGDOM OF LIFE THAN A VEGETABLE. A vegetable earns its living one ray of sunlight at a time. Vegetables don't hide, hunt, sneak, prowl, gamble, brag, or flirt. Once their working lives end they offer themselves to us naked in their bins, with no boastful labels, no gimmicks, no enticements.

The honest vegetable deserves a promotion from side dish to main dish. Yet I understand your lack of enthusiasm. Like an online dating profile, vegetables look perfect from a distance. Their images are beautiful and their characteristics are impressive. But when you get face to face with that vegetable, it's so dull it could put you to sleep during a hurricane. Don't despair—in a few pages I'll teach you how to meet the vegetables of your dreams. First, though, we need to correct two pervasive misconceptions. First: The beneficial effects of vegetables *cannot* be distilled. Second: Fruits and vegetables *are not equally beneficial* for weight loss.

"Superfoods" and Supplements, Snake Oil for the 21st Century

Think about how often you see a nutrient, together with its parent food, lauded for its health-promoting effects. It's hard not to want to put some faith in those claims—who wouldn't want to get healthy by eating chocolate and drinking wine or by popping a supplement and munching on a trendy, high-status "superfood"?

That wishful thinking has thoroughly wormed its way into public consciousness: "Vegetables are really good for you, so their 'magical' nutrients just need to be extracted, added to, or processed into something delicious or convenient, and presto—perfect health!"

The food and supplement industries happily cater to our wish for easy solutions. They fund studies on micronutrients (vitamins, minerals, and phytonutrients) found in plants. Any favorable outcome results in a blitz of advertising or a public relations campaign.

Their studies aren't outright fraudulent, but they *are* misleading. They focus on foods with high profit margins (e.g., chocolate, wine, coffee, nuts) and foods for which the supply can be controlled, like imported foods, foods that need processing, or foods that can be processed into supplements. And, it should be noted, the studies that reveal no benefit aren't publicized.

Promoting nutrition in this way contributes to the profitable illusion that nutrients are rare and health is mysterious, complicated, and elusive. No missing magical nutrient holds the key to your health. Nutrients are abundant. Deficiencies are easily met by common, inexpensive foods. There are no superfoods. There is no hierarchy of plants: all edible plants contain a variety of beneficial nutrients.

The fact that cheap, unprocessed commodities like beans, cabbage, and carrots are rarely promoted for their benefits isn't a measure of their relative nutritional value. They're ignored because they represent a slim profit margin and minimal opportunity to corner a market. (You can't patent a carrot, but you could patent "Sunshine Carotene Essence.") The paradox in all this magical thinking is that **unprocessed vegetables,** with their stomach-filling structure, are the only magic pill for weight loss. As I note in my discussion of starches and calories in the last two chapters, *structure is meaning.*

Don't fall for the gimmicks — "superfoods," green drinks, powders, capsules, pills, and supplements. While it's possible that a few of these products might offer modest benefits for certain health conditions (check with your doctor or dietitian), most offer nothing special and *none* are effective for weight loss.

We haven't come very far in 130 years.

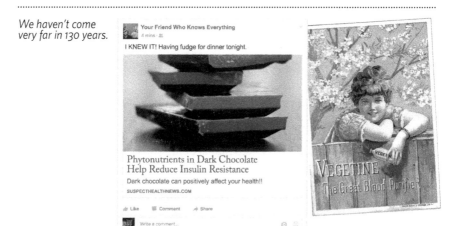

Dad's Berries (The Grass Is Greener...)

One summer day I was visiting my parents and noticed a small bag of dried goji berries on the kitchen counter. I popped a few in my mouth. They were chewy and sweet, like candy. Minutes later I had eaten half the bag. I looked at the nutrition label to check the damage (*Yikes! More than 400 calories!*), then noticed something even more shocking: the price. I teased my normally bargain-oriented father, "Hey, Dad — why did you spend 12 dollars on a tiny bag of goji berries?" He answered, "Well, they're a superfood from China. I read a study that they have phytonutrients that boost the immune system." "Dad," I said, "You have three blueberry bushes in the front yard, a back yard full of growing vegetables, and a fridge full of store-bought vegetables. You're *swimming* in phytonutrients!" Maybe a clever business in China is even now making a mint selling its latest exotic superfood: dried Maryland blueberries.

The irony is that my father is an accomplished horticulturist, and a journalist who wrote the organic gardening column for *The Washington Post* for decades. If even he enthusiastically fell for a common marketing trick, can anyone — including our highly educated media — be immune?

Señor Zanahoria & Señora Pera

"Eat your fruits and vegetables."
"Two cups a day of fruits and vegetables"
"Make half your plate fruits and vegetables."

Public health officials, doctors, and dietitians all repeat the same messages. Fruits and vegetables sit together in the store and we always talk about them together. You might think, "That's okay, it's one or the other...right?" Unfortunately, that's *not* the case. Because fruits are sweet and don't require preparation time, most people respond enthusiastically to upping their fruit intake but conveniently forget about the veggies. **Fruits and vegetables have entirely distinct effects on weight.**

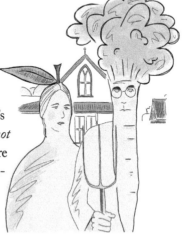

In the healthcare field we use the nutritional definition of fruits and vegetables, not the botanical. While a botanist would say peppers and cucumbers are fruits because they grow out of the flower's ovary, we call them vegetables because they meet our nutritional definition: low in sugars and calories, high in fiber and complex carbohydrates. In contrast, fruits are high in simple carbohydrates (sugars) and contain moderate amounts of calories and fiber.

Fruits, Veggies, and Your Gut

Vegetables average four times more fiber per calorie than fruits. Whole grains, whose high-fiber attributes are heavily promoted, average only one-eighth as much fiber per calorie as vegetables. The differences matter because **fiber** helps with weight loss via many effects:

1. It increases the weight and volume of food, which makes us feel more full.

2. It slows down the digestion process. A slower digestion speed increases satiety and slows the release of energy from food, helping to keep our blood sugars within a healthy range.

3. It acts as a training partner for the muscles. The workout starts in the mouth where fiber increases chewing time. Chewing burns calories and makes us eat slower. A similar process continues in the digestive tract, where fiber increases the number and strength of muscle contractions.

4. Flexing intestinal muscles burn calories while communicating a feeling of fullness to the brain.

Fruits are digested rapidly, containing mostly water, simple carbohydrates/ sugars, and less fiber. Most importantly for weight loss, the divide in sugars and fiber impacts calories. Fruits average 60 calories per serving, while vegetables average only 25 calories per serving.

Calorie content per 100 grams / 3.5 ounces

The equivalent of a small apple, 4-6 strawberries, an average-sized carrot, or a large bell pepper.

Fruits	cal.	Veggies	cal.
Watermelon	26	Lettuce	17
Plum	46	Mushrooms	18
Orange	53	Bell Pepper	20
Apple	56	Spinach	23
Cherries	70	Cabbage	25
Mango	70	Cauliflower	27
Strawberries	77	Broccoli	29
Banana	95	Carrot	40
Dates	281	Onion	41

In sum, **vegetables are essential** for weight loss while **fruits are neutral.** In moderation (two to four servings per day), fruits can be a useful player in a weight loss diet, particularly when used as a substitute for sweets.

The Vegetable of Your Dreams, an Owner's Manual

I teach college nutrition courses and when we delve into the section on vegetables I always hear from the immigrants in my class. With a diplomatic tone they say they love their new life in the USA but the supermarkets are disappointing: the meats have little taste, the fruits are bland, and the vegetables are particularly disappointing. These students come from countries where the markets have fresh food delivered daily from nearby farms. In rustic stalls the butcher snaps the chicken's neck and plucks its feathers for a customer; the fishmonger happily cuts the fish open to reveal the still-beating heart. American capitalism has done an enviable job at creating competitive markets that result in low-cost, high-quality goods, but has not been able to replicate this success with raw agricultural products — particularly vegetables.

Conventional: Convenience Conquers All

Imagine if cars had no brand names. You'd pick out a car based on the size, shape, and color but wouldn't know who made it or where it was made. There would be no incentive on manufacturers' part to make a high-quality automobile because their product wouldn't be traceable. Similarly, agricultural products are mostly faceless commodities. The farmer who takes great care to cultivate succulent squash is paid the same as one who puts in little effort. If you happen to love the tomatoes at a grocery store one day, you can't go back to the produce manager a few days later and ask "What farm did you get Tuesday's tomatoes from? I would like those same tomatoes again."

The majority of conventional raw agricultural products end up as animal feed or go to food processing plants for use in packaged foods. Conventional farming is focused on producing blank slates; like stainless steel cars rolling down the assembly line for layers of paint and racing stripes, the crops wait for their personality to be applied in the sauces, sweeteners, salt, and chemical flavor additives of the food industry.

It is not only a question of profit. Conventional produce is bred and selected for pleasing, uniform appearance; the ability to produce profitable, high-yield harvests; and the durability to weather the beatings that come with storage and transport over long distances. Conventional seeds are bred for similar agronomic realities and to align with the mechanics of production: growth to a uniform height, position of edible portions on the plant, consistent harvest schedule, and the ability to withstand particular pesticide applications.

Small-Scale Surprises: Flavor First

Prioritizing low price over taste is an obstacle to falling in love with vegetables. Fortunately, there are alternative vendors that curate selections of vegetables based on flavor and freshness: health food stores, ethnic markets (particularly Asian and Latino), and my favorite, community-supported agriculture. A CSA is a farm that sells shares of its harvest: members buy local, seasonal food directly from the farmer. Comparable to buying stock from a company or joining a fantasy football league, buying through a CSA is almost a form of small-scale gambling—something else to discuss around the water cooler on Mondays. *("Have you ever seen that kind of purple squash? Those sweet-meat pumpkins were amazing!")* Seasonal yields vary; some years might feature a bumper crop of your favorite asparagus while other years deliver a small mountain of beets. In addition to the edible dividends, many CSAs hold farm-based events. You might get to pick your own raspberries, learn how to can tomatoes or make pickles, or milk a goat. As the movement grows, more CSAs are expanding their offerings to include fresh meats, culinary herbs, pickled vegetables, and even cooking classes.

Branding Raw Agricultural Products

CSAs have incentive to produce the highest-quality goods because they are meeting their customers in person. As part of this more intimate relationship, CSA farmers are redefining the market by producing the first brands for what have generally been regarded as unbranded commodities. Their heirloom varieties with boutique-ish titles reflect this. (It's not a handbag, it's a Gucci; these are not green beans, they are Blue Lake pole beans.) Unlike handbags, however, the differences are deeper than the names.

The future is likely to see a continuation of this trend with CSAs organizing to regulate the branding of their products. They might gather to create standards for different varieties and create metrics for qualities such as taste, texture, and nutrient composition. Speaking of nutrient composition, conventional produce is picked before it is ripe so that it can ripen during the long transport and storage process. This early picking affects more than flavor. The longer a plant remains in the ground, the longer the roots can pull up soil minerals; and with the extra time, the plant synthesizes more vitamins and phytonutrients. CSAs pick produce within a day or two of bringing them to customers, maximizing nutrition and flavor.

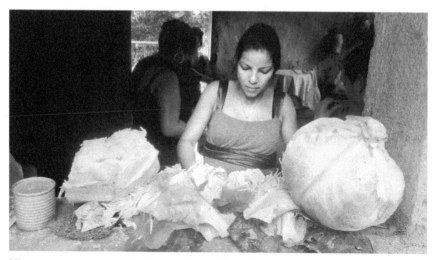

Nicaraguans grow an abundance of vegetables, but on average they eat less than a cup of vegetables a day. Cabbage is the most common because it is cheap, easy to prepare, can keep well for well more than a week with no refrigeration. Most often it is eaten as a side salad, shredded with a little tomato and carrot, and tossed with lime or vinegar and salt. (*El Jícaro, Departamento de Nueva Segovia*)

A Bushel of Veggie Options

While fresh CSA veggies are the gold standard, we need many options for vegetables if they are to make up half of our meals. Don't turn your nose up to frozen, dehydrated, and canned veggies. The two most common reasons people don't eat enough veggies are taste and convenience. Here we address those two obstacles:

1 **Marinate!** There are dozens of delicious low-calorie marinades you can make. Let your veggies soak for an hour or so, and then bake, grill, or sauté. (The Appendix has a few recipes—see page 205.)

2 **Experiment with textures**. Use a food processor to shred beets, celery, onions, scallions, and carrots for salads, stir-fries, and stews.

3 **Sprout!** Sprouting converts seeds, grains, and legumes into low calorie-density vegetables. Electric sprouters are easy to use and inexpensive, but you can sprout with common kitchen items as well.

4 **Ferment!** Common fermented vegetables are pickles, kimchi, and sauerkraut. You can find many others at ethnic markets (Korean, Russian), health food stores, CSAs, and farmers' markets. You can also easily make them at home. To get started, check out the website of Sandor Katz, guru of fermentation.

Visit wildfermentation.com

5   **Look for a fungus among us.** Although botanically not a vegetable, the low calorie density of mushrooms allows them to be categorized with vegetables. They have a meaty taste and are packed with nutrients. They're also easy to cultivate at home with kits (available at health food stores and online). Mycologist Paul Stamets' website has good resources.   Visit fungi.com

6   **Buy pre-cut, pre-washed vegetables** and salad greens to save time.

7   **Try sea vegetables.** Dulse and wakame are delicious in soups or cooked with legumes. Some other seaweeds work well with salads and meat dishes. Sea vegetables contain a wide array of minerals and add flavor with almost no calories. There is even a pasta-like product made out of the common seaweed called kelp.

8   **Smell your way to health with herbs.** If your vegetables smell fragrant you are more likely to enjoy their flavor at every meal. Store-bought bunches of fresh herbs can be expensive, so buy herb plants for the kitchen windowsill and add in a few leaves every time you prepare veggies.

9   **Maintain a "salad bar" in your refrigerator.** Keep a few storage containers filled with cut up greens and veggies. They'll be ready at a moment's notice to make a salad, add to a sandwich, or prepare as a side dish.

10 **Cook or marinate with wine, whiskey, or rum.** The alcohol burns off— and with it the calories—but the flavor remains.

11 **Experiment with dehydrated vegetables.** These veggies used to be just for the camping crowd, but cooks on the go have discovered they are an effortless way to get more veggies into soups and stews.

12 **Check out the frozen-foods section of your grocery store.** You'll find a few healthy options hiding next to the ice cream: staples like spinach and okra and tasty vegetable mixes. Look for blends with names like California, Asian, Mediterranean, and Stir-Fry.

13 **Make use of canned veggies.** When fresh tomatoes aren't in season, canned tomatoes are a great shortcut to making pasta sauces and marinades, and a great addition to soups, stews, and chilies. Other useful canned vegetables include spinach, turnips, beets, pumpkin, asparagus, and collard greens.

14 **Don't forget about glass-jar veggies.** You'll find these in the same supermarket aisle as relishes, olives, and other condiments. A step up from canned, glass-jar veggies offer convenience. Just make sure they're packed in water, not oil. My favorites are roasted red peppers, strained tomatoes, artichoke hearts, hearts of palm, and green beans.

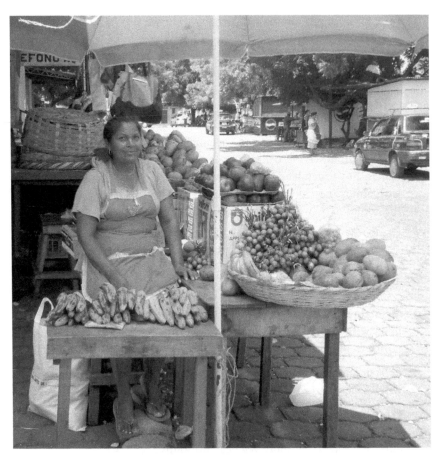

In Nicaragua, like much of the developing world, few people eat canned or frozen fruits and vegetables. In part this is because refrigeration is expensive. Most Nicas buy fresh fruits and vegetables from the myriad markets and street vendors. Cities typically also have a thriving system of pickup-truck-based entrepreneurs (in smaller towns vendors have horse- or donkey-drawn carts) who follow regular daily routes selling produce and staples like beans, corn, and rice. (*Managua*)

CHAPTER 7

Protein

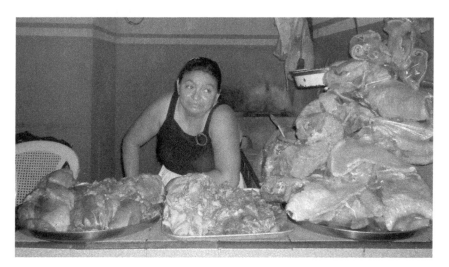

A surfeit of protein. Marta sells fried pork skin and raw kidneys and liver. Often, meat is not refrigerated in Nicaragua and inexpensive organ meats and ground meat are common. The more expensive cuts of meat are exported. (*Managua*)

FEELING BLUE? WANT TO GAIN MUSCLE? LOSE WEIGHT? KICK YOUR CRAVINGS? All you need to do is double down on protein. Ah, if only it were so easy. Protein is the overrated rock star in the world of nutrition—the most complex member of the power trio macronutrient band, both in its structure and in the multitude of physiological roles it plays. While protein is essential for health, most people worry too much about it without understanding its role.

It's hardly an overnight sensation as a celebrity. In preindustrial societies consuming animals was a sign of status; the hunter was the hero of the tribe. In feudal, agricultural societies royalty feasted on game while peasants ate grains and legumes. Even today, particularly in the developing world, eating animals signifies wealth. Low-protein diets have been associated with physical and even psychological weakness.

Some of protein's prestige is deserved. When our health is compromised—by conditions such as AIDS, cancer, surgery, broken bones, or burns—our protein needs double or even triple as our bodies utilize it to repair tissue and fortify our immune system.

Macronutrients are the three nutrients that contain calories: carbohydrates, fat, and protein.

With all that in mind, it may not be a surprise that Americans consume, on average, about twice the recommended daily allowance (RDA) set by the government.[1] Perhaps the medical role and historical scarcity of animal protein have influenced us. For much of history it was hard to get enough, and we now default to overemphasizing what was once limited. Or it could be that protein's role in muscle synthesis has led us to the common misconception that when you eat protein, it goes straight into your muscles. This is the thinking behind half-baked ideas like "cake goes right to your thighs" or "beer goes straight to your belly." While it is true that protein deficiency will swiftly decimate your vitality, an excess has no benefits. Excess calories from any source are converted into fat all over your body, including bellies and thighs.

In this chapter we will demythologize protein and answer the key questions regarding protein's role in weight loss: How much protein do we need? Are there risks associated with eating too much or too little protein? What are the best protein sources?

Soldiers, Babies, and Everyone in Between

Since protein is essential for the function of our immune system and for the physical structure and maintenance of our muscles, many organizations have studied and set standards for protein intake.

The USDA sets the RDA for protein at 0.36 grams per pound. That works out to just over one-third of your body weight in grams [*weight in pounds* × 0.36, or *weight in kilograms* × 0.8]. To illustrate, the recommendation for a 150-pound adult is 54 grams per day (or 216 calories—just over 10 percent of calories assuming a 2000-calorie-per-day diet).

The U.S. military calculates intake for active-duty soldiers at 13 percent of daily calories. Meals Ready to Eat (MREs), the portable rations provided to active-duty soldiers, use the 13 percent figure.

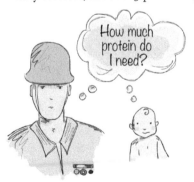

How much protein do I need?

Babies need protein to build organ tissues such as the heart, lungs, liver, kidneys, and rapidly growing muscles. Babies thrive on only breast milk, which is a mere 7 percent protein (the remainder is 53 percent fat and 40 percent carbohydrate). Infant formula, which is modeled on breast milk, is usually about 9 percent protein.

One gram of protein is approximately four calories.

How about athletes? A lifestyle that includes sufficient physical activity to build a toned, muscled physique can be maintained with the standard RDA for protein. If your goals include increasing muscle size and strength, then your protein needs increase. This works out to between 60 and 75 grams (240–300 calories) of protein for an active 150-pound adult and up to 120 grams (480 calories) for a competitive athlete. Keep in mind that muscle weighs more than fat, so a muscle-building program will slow weight loss. However, it is well worth the few extra pounds. Muscle weight looks trim, hard, and fit. More importantly, muscles, even at rest, burn more calories than fat. This metabolic boost gives even a modest weight lifter (twice-weekly sessions of an hour each are enough to make an impact) a permanent edge with keeping weight off.

The National Strength and Conditioning Association recommends that active people consume 0.4 to 0.6 grams of protein per pound of body weight, while competitive athletes can go up to 0.8 grams per pound.

Can You Eat Too Much or Too Little Protein?

To maximize weight loss, dieters need to eat a moderate portion of protein with every meal. Protein's complex structure takes time to break down into its digestible parts, the amino acids. This lengthy process occurs in the stomach. Since little happens with fats and carbohydrates in the stomach, we need protein to give us the satisfying feeling of a working stomach. However, there is no need for protein neurosis. You can be a healthy and successful dieter both barely meeting requirements and eating up to double the requirements. The dangers lie only in the extremes.

Deficits: To avoid protein deficiency, which can decrease immune system functioning and result in loss of muscle tissue, the World Health Organization recommends a minimum intake of 5 percent of your daily calories as protein. On a 2,000-calorie diet this would be about 25 grams per day, or 100 calories. Protein deficiency is rare in developed countries, where diets typically triple or even quadruple this amount.

Excess: If protein is satiating and nutritious, isn't more better? This alluring notion leads many to assume we can wolf down all the protein we desire. But extra calories from any source become fat, and in protein's case the consequences of excess don't stop at weight gain. Protein, unlike fat and carbohydrates, contains nitrogen. Nitrogen, when unbound from protein, is toxic. When we consume excess protein, unbound nitrogen is released. It is removed by the liver and processed into urea by the kidneys, where it becomes a component in urine. Patients with liver or kidney diseases are put on low-protein diets because excess nitrogen can tax those organs to the point of failure. Excess protein also causes excretion of calcium in the urine, contributing to poor bone health. If we ate an appropriate quantity of protein, we would likely have lower incidences of liver, kidney, and bone disease. The upper limit of safe protein intake depends on many factors including age, activity, protein source, and current health status and is an area of ongoing research. The general scientific consensus is that consistently eating more than twice the RDA is where the possibility of negative consequences begins.

Three Common Reasons We Overestimate Protein Needs

1 All protein estimates, including the official recommendations discussed in the previous paragraphs, are calculated for a body composition that falls in the healthy range.[2] Consider the two Davids pictured below: "Slim D," 150 pounds in his 20s; and the same fellow, "Heavy D," a few years later at 200 pounds, with 50 pounds of excess fat. Heavy D's protein needs remain unchanged. Excess body fat does not utilize protein so it does not increase our protein needs.

2 The body prefers not to burn protein for energy. Unlike fat and carbohydrates, protein is conserved. Worn-out proteins are recycled by the liver and reused. There is an exception, however: on low-carbohydrate diets the body burns protein (as well as fat) for energy. Since the primary store of protein is our muscles, people who follow low-carbohydrate diets can inadvertently lose muscle.[3]

3 Protein is not only available in animal flesh. Dairy, legumes, nuts, seeds, starches, and vegetables have protein. There is even a little protein in some fruits, particularly those with edible seeds, such as strawberries and blackberries. Many vegetables contain protein, calorie per calorie, in amounts comparable to traditional protein sources. You might assume that roasted, skinless chicken breast is a great protein source, and it is—a 100 calorie, two-ounce portion contains 20 grams. Steak (depending on the cut) contains a little less protein, about 5 to 10 grams per 100 calories. In comparison, 100 calories of spinach contains 13 grams of protein while 100 calories of broccoli contains 6.8 grams.

Different weights, same protein needs

Protein and the Sober Plate

Don't break out a calculator—you don't need to count your protein grams. There is a wide range of options for healthy protein intake; neither deficiency nor excess is possible on the Food Sobriety diet. At every meal one-quarter of your plate will feature a palm-sized portion (roughly three to four ounces) of animal protein, or four to eight ounces of legumes, or one serving of dairy (size is dependent on choice). This portion will provide 10 to 30 grams of protein and between 75 and 150 calories per meal.

Below are two days worth of Sober Plate-style meals with their protein grams calculated. Both easily exceed the RDA of 54 grams for a 150-pound adult (and this is without counting snacks).

Conventional Menu

BREAKFAST
2-egg omelet (14g) with ½ cup peppers (1g),
½ cup of asparagus (2g), and 1 cup of rice (5g)

LUNCH
One 4-ounce extra-lean turkey burger (30g) with bun (3g),
lettuce, tomato, onion (1g), and 1 cup of sauerkraut (1g)

DINNER
4 ounces of baked chicken (28g) with 1 cup of
roasted broccoli (4g) and 1 cup of corn (4.5g)

Total Protein: 93.5 grams

Vegan Version

BREAKFAST
Breakfast burrito — flour tortilla (5.5g) with 3/4 cup of black beans (11g),
½ cup of mixed veggies (2.5g), and ¼ cup of salsa (2.5g)

LUNCH
1 cup of cooked spinach (6g), 1 medium bowl of lentil soup (15g),
and 1 cup of wild rice (6.5g)

DINNER
1 cup of mushrooms (3.5g), 1 cup of roasted cauliflower (3g),
12 oz. of vegetarian chili (18g), and a 6-oz. baked potato (5g)

Total Protein: 78.5 grams

Sources, Part One: Plant-Based Proteins

"One farmer says to me, 'You cannot live on vegetable food solely, for it furnishes nothing to make bones with'; and so he religiously devotes a part of his day to supplying his system with the raw material of bones; walking all the while he talks behind his oxen, which, with vegetable-made bones, jerk him and his lumbering plow along in spite of every obstacle."

HENRY DAVID THOREAU, *WALDEN*, 1854

The Flexitarian Approach

You can take Thoreau's point quite a distance. Similarly fantastic musculature, strength, and stamina can be observed in a variety of herbivores that consume well under 20 percent of their calories as protein: horses, deer, buffalo, kangaroos, and our large-primate cousins such as silverback and lowland gorillas.

Because weight loss is achievable via a spectrum of diets, it makes sense to be open toward varying, even opposing, dietary philosophies. While the following pages provide a rationale for substituting plant-based proteins for animal-based proteins, I am not making the case for veganism. Rather, I am recognizing that many of the most effective diets for weight loss are plant-based diets, or, as they are often called, **flexitarian** diets.

One of the leading advocates of the plant-based diet is Dr. Colin Campbell, author of *The China Study*. In one of the most comprehensive research projects ever undertaken, Campbell, in collaboration with Cornell University and the Chinese Academy of Preventive Medicine, studied the diets of a large cross section of Chinese society for several decades. The conclusion is compelling:

> "People who ate the most animal-based foods got the most chronic disease ... People who ate the most plant-based foods were the healthiest and tended to avoid chronic disease."[4]

The China Study also concluded that diets with high percentages of animal protein increase cancer risk, while those with low percentages of animal protein or more plant proteins lower cancer risk. Campbell emphasizes that dairy products, despite their reputation of being healthier than meat, share a similar mix of fats and proteins, and carry the same health impact.

While the explanations behind Campbell's results will be debated for years, one certainty is that animals' position at the top of the food chain has consequences. All the agricultural chemicals that are used in producing animal feed, including the pollutants in the water supply, reach far greater concentration in animal flesh and dairy products than in any other food source. Similarly, a significant percentage of seafood has traces of heavy metals, mercury, and other pollutants. To minimize your exposure you can choose organic meats and dairy with the lowest fat—the most potent toxins accumulate in the fat, not the protein. For the safest seafood check the Monterey Bay Aquarium's Seafood Watch website.   **Visit www.seafoodwatch.org**

A Caloric Argument for a Plant-Based Diet

When we calculate protein calories we use the value of four calories per gram, although that number is only an average of the calories available from different foods. The original research into the energy contained in varying foods is summarized well in *Why Calories Count*, by Marion Nestle and Malden Nesheim. Protein from animals (meats, eggs, and dairy) yields 4.25 to 4.35 calories per gram. Protein from plants (grains, legumes, vegetables, and fruits) yields 2.9 to 3.7 calories per gram. Calories from fat are 9 per gram for animal-based foods and only 8.35 for plant-based foods.[5] This information relates to how we calculate calories using a bomb calorimeter, discussed in Chapter 4.

That we assimilate fewer calories from plants is likely due to the fact that the fiber and resistant starch in plant foods impedes full absorption of the calories while, at the same time, causing the digestive tract to burn more calories in the process (increasing the thermic effect). For instance, the protein contained in legumes only yields 3.2 calories per gram while the protein in meat yields 4.2. The protein in legumes needs to be "mined out" by the digestive tract—removed from a matrix of fiber and water.

Eating 100 grams of animal protein per day yields 425 to 435 calories, while eating 100 grams of plant protein yields 290 to 370 calories. If an additional 50 grams from animal fat is added, the meat eater gets 450 more calories. If 50 grams of plant fat is added, the vegetarian gains only 418 additional calories. These cumulative additions can make the difference between gaining or losing several pounds a year and partially explain why vegetarians weigh less, on average, than omnivores.

This difference also explains why animal protein is ranked as higher quality than plant protein. Nutritional science, having been traditionally concerned with lack of growth (not excess growth) has always defined protein quality in terms of weight gain. **Protein quality** is the efficiency at which proteins can be absorbed and digested from the diet; animal proteins are higher quality because they promote faster weight gain.

Plant-Based Proteins

For those seeking the benefit from the inclusion of at least some meat-free meals, the two best options follow.

Legumes

Also called pulses, **legumes** include all varieties of beans, lentils, and peas. They have plenty of protein and almost no fat, and their high fiber and water content result in a long-lasting satiety. Legumes also have a high percentage of resistant starch. They are the least expensive protein and are a snap to prepare. The Academy of Nutrition and Dietetics recommends that vegans consume legumes at every meal. Similarly, for weight loss, most meatless meals should contain legumes. Some tips to keep in mind:

- **Soak:** Soaking legumes before cooking aids digestion. Soaking time varies by variety—anywhere from 20 minutes to several hours.

- **Season:** Methods for eliminating digestive discomfort and gas include cooking legumes with any of the following: bay leaves, kombu (a tasty seaweed, available in Asian markets and health food stores), garlic, ginger, and cumin.

- **Sprout:** Sprouting your legumes for a few days prior to cooking increases digestibility, may aid weight loss (it increases water content and lowers the caloric density), and results in a light, creamy flavor. You can cook the legumes the moment a sprout appears or you can wait. A legume with a long sprout needs less cooking time than one with a short sprout. When a legume is fully sprouted it can be eaten raw.

The only exceptions to the legume rule are peanuts and soybeans. While most legumes derive less than one percent of their calories from fat, these two come in at over 20 percent. The high caloric density means vigorous portion control is needed if these foods are to be a regular part of the diet.

Calories per
1/2 cup (cooked)

Black beans........105

Soybeans.............155

Dry-roasted
peanuts.................413

Chapter 5 explains resistant starch.
Although nuts and seeds contain protein, they draw the majority of their calories from fat. They are discussed in **Chapter 8.**

A Few Favorite Meat Substitutes

Beyond Meat	This line of soy- and pea-based meat substitutes gets high marks for mimicking the look, taste, and texture of meat. The Grilled Strips are popular: at 120 calories and 20 grams of protein per three-ounce serving they are also a great fit for weight loss.
Gardenburger	One of the older lines of vegetarian products with many tasty options.
MorningStar Farms	Their "Grillers" burgers are delicious and nutritious.
Homemade	Veggie burgers are easy and fun to make. Check the recipes in the Appendix.

Meat Substitutes

Vegetarian meat substitutes have made great strides since the 1980s, when a glob of cereal crumbs glued together with egg yolk passed as a veggie burger. The new meat substitutes have some distinct advantages:

- They're convenient. You can pop them into a toaster oven or skillet and eat moments later.
- Most are lower in calories than animal proteins and many are high in fiber.
- The simple tastes and familiar shapes are a hit with kids.

You can't assume that meat substitutes will help with weight loss—some do and some don't. The vegetarian market includes plenty of customers who are not at all concerned with calories. Ignore the health claims on the packaging. Look at the nutrition facts and especially at the serving size. A good guideline is (per three- to four-ounce serving): 80 to 150 calories, fewer than five grams of fat, and more than two grams of fiber.

Sources, Part Two: Animal Protein

Five Meaty Considerations

Fat: Ideally, the meat you eat should have about one gram of fat or less per ounce. Don't focus on the type of meat. For instance, turkey is generally lower in fat than pork, but you can find both very lean cuts of pork and fatty cuts of turkey. If you prefer higher-fat cuts, then the portion size needs to decrease proportionately.

Confusing labels: Ground raw beef is a classic example. Labeled as "90% lean," it actually draws half of its calories from fat. The labels relate to the **weight of the fat** in the uncooked product. The "96% lean" version is better, but the calories from fat are still higher than you might expect (about 32 percent).

To do the math yourself, ignore the percentage. Look at the label and compare "total calories" with "calories from fat." Check the same part of the label when you purchase seafood. While most seafood is quite low in fat be cautious with cold-water fish and frozen seafood products (breaded shrimp or pre-seasoned fish fillets); their calories quickly become hamburger-esque.

Nutrition Facts
Serving Size 4 oz. (112g)
Servings per container varied

Amount Per Serving
Calories 200   Calories from Fat 100

% Daily Value*
Total Fat 11g   17%

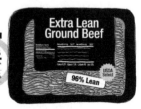

Lean Ground Beef

90% Lean

$$100 \div 200 = 0.50$$
"90% lean" actually means 50% fat.

Water content: The water content of food gives it bulk and volume, which contributes to feeling full. For instance, a 150-calorie serving of turkey leg contains more water, and thus volume, than a 150-calorie serving of turkey in the form of a few slim deli slices or a handful of turkey jerky "niblets."

Nutrition Facts
Serving Size 4 oz. (112g)
Servings per container varied

Amount Per Serving
Calories 140   Calories from Fat 45

% Daily Value*
Total Fat 5g   7%

Extra Lean Ground Beef

96% Lean

$$45 \div 140 = 0.32$$
"96% lean" actually means 32% fat.

Preparation: Are you adding calories in the cooking or were calories added in the processing? Typical culprits are cooking oils, sugary glazes, and oily marinades. For example, when you're dieting it's better to eat poached eggs than scrambled eggs, since you need oil or butter for the scrambled version.

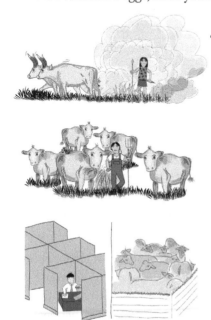

Quality: Animals essentially come in three "brands"—wild, pasture raised, and conventional (or "modern"). Modern animals, kept in feedlots and fed mostly grains and soy, are two to eight times higher in fat than the lean wild game our ancestors ate. Animals are like us. If they eat heavy diets and lack activity they lose muscle and gain fat. In between these extremes are the pasture-raised animals that our great-grandparents grew up on. In fact, the pre-World War II style of animal husbandry is now making a comeback because of both animal welfare and ecological concerns. Aficionados praise pasture-raised meat as lower in fat and richer in flavor than feedlot meat.

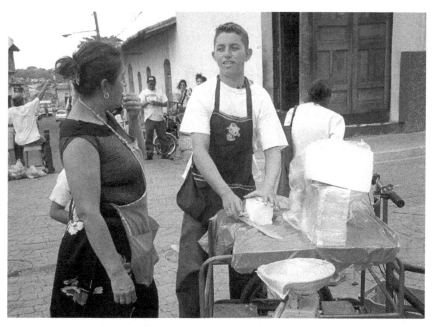

Sixteen-year-old Hernando sells cheese from his bicycle cart. Cheese provides the high calorie and nutrient density of meat at a fraction of the cost. In a developing country like Nicaragua this makes cheese a valued commodity. *(Leon)*

Dairy: Politics, Recommendations, and Labels

I saved dairy for last, as it is a complex and controversial category. The human species, *Homo sapiens*, is estimated to be approximately four hundred thousand years old. Humans domesticated dairy animals about ten thousand years ago. Three-quarters of the world's population does not consume dairy. From both historical and global perspectives dairy is not an essential food group for humans; it is an optional food group.

Our government's classification of dairy as essential is worth reconsidering:

1. We are the only mammals that continue to consume dairy past infancy. Dairy is an essential food only for infants (breast milk or a dairy-based infant formula).

2. Most non-Caucasians lack the enzyme to digest dairy products.

3. The calorie density of dairy products can contribute to excess weight.

Though controversial as a food group, dairy earned its prominent role in public health guidelines through legitimate means. Throughout most of the 20th century our government faced far more problems with underweight populations living in poverty than with obesity. Dairy, with its potent weight-gain properties, was an effective commodity to distribute to the needy. Public health officials, in particular, valued cheese. Cheese is less expensive than meat, takes longer to spoil than milk, and packs a ton of calories into a compact and popular form. Cheese was delivered to the poor via a variety of government programs including subsidized student lunches and welfare. During the 20th century dairy products did an outstanding job of ensuring that several generations of impoverished Americans were able to avoid stunted growth, malnutrition, and hunger.

The dairy trade's successful partnership with government grew over the decades until it became one of the most politically connected industries in the country. The industry now funds—via universities, hospitals, and research foundations—thousands of studies to promote dairy's benefits. Their reach extends to government groups and health organizations, including the Academy of Nutrition and Dietetics, the U.S. Department of Agriculture, and the U.S. Department of Health and Human Services. The end result is that the industry maintains a strong influence in determining dietary recommendations and agricultural policy.

Dairy and Bones

One of the chief rationales for dairy's inclusion as an essential food group comes from the belief that it is required for bone health. However, humans who lived before the advent of dairy farming had bone health that varied little from our own. The percentage of the world population that does not consume dairy shows no evidence of poorer bone health than the 25 percent that does. Many other environmental and nutritional factors affect bone health, and it is easy to build and maintain healthy bones with or without dairy.

You do need calcium-rich foods for bone health, *but consuming calcium does not guarantee it*. For the body to incorporate calcium into bones it needs:

- **Activity:** When you use your bones, your body responds by sending bone-building nutrients, including calcium, to your bones. All activity helps, but weight-bearing activities (such as weight lifting, walking, hiking, jogging, climbing stairs, tennis, and dancing) are most effective.

- Other bone-building **nutrients**: magnesium, boron, zinc, and vitamins D and K.

In the absence of those factors the body can't use calcium. It deals with the excess by eliminating calcium in urine, which can cause the buildup that becomes kidney stones; and circulating extra calcium in the blood, where it can attach itself to artery walls, weakening them and contributing to heart disease. Other things that weaken bone health include excess coffee (drinking more than two cups a day); excess phosphorus (sources with the highest content are animal products, dairy, and dark-colored soft drinks); excess salt (more than two grams per day); smoking; and some medications, such as synthetic thyroid hormones, steroids, aluminum-containing antacids, some diuretics, and some antibiotics.

Recommendations and Labels

Having considered dairy's role in our national history and in our bones, let's consider the bigger biological picture. What is the purpose of milk on this planet? Milk is among the evolutionary adaptations that turned a branch of reptiles into mammals. Instead of laying lots of eggs and hoping that some of the hapless tiny newborns would survive, the strategy of the mammals was to have fewer babies and invest more energy in each infant. Two of the "investment strategies" were to grow the fetus inside the body and to nurture the helpless newborn with a potent growth serum. Milk's role is to add weight and do it quickly. Dairy is a powerful, transformative food, magical in its potency. It is an ideal food for underweight individuals — particularly youth — but it has a limited role for overweight adults.

The U.S. government's official nutrition planner (choosemyplate.gov) has five food groups: grains, vegetables, fruits, dairy, and protein foods. The Food Sobriety diet counts dairy as a protein because it provides the same amount of protein as legumes, which all food classification systems count as a pro-

The U.S. government recommends adults consume three servings of dairy a day. A serving is:
- 8 ounces of milk or yogurt, or
- 1.5 ounces of cheese (about the size of a 9-volt battery).

A serving of legumes is four ounces. Both legumes and dairy provide about 8 grams of protein per serving.

tein. There are a few dairy products (e.g., butter, cream, cream cheese, and high-fat cheeses like brie and Camembert) that don't contain significant protein. Because they are so high in fat they are considered fats, not proteins, in all food systems.

If you want to keep dairy in your daily diet you have options: 1) consume whole-fat dairy and be vigilant about portion size; 2) consume low-fat dairy and enjoy 20-percent-larger portions than full fat; 3) consume nonfat dairy and be able to have about twice as much as full fat. Is it necessary to go to the "extreme" of nonfat dairy — isn't low fat good enough? Whether to choose the richer flavor of the higher-fat product or the stomach-filling volume of the alternative is up to you.

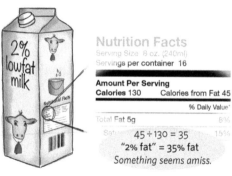

Nutrition Facts
Serving Size 8 oz. (240ml)
Servings per container 16

Amount Per Serving
Calories 130   Calories from Fat 45

% Daily Value*

Total Fat 5g   8%

Satur   45 ÷ 130 = 35   15%
"2% fat" = 35% fat
Something seems amiss.

Regardless of your choice, you must learn to *decipher the misleading labels* used for dairy products. For example: "2% low fat milk" means that 2 percent of the weight of the milk is from fat. This is the equivalent of labeling a 12-ounce can of Coke as 9 percent sugar because the 35 grams of sugar in the Coke account for 9 percent of the weight (390 grams). Can you imagine the outrage if the beverage industry started labeling sugar the way the dairy industry labels fat? It's not just milk. All dairy products are labeled with a percentage that describes the contribution fat makes to the total weight (not calories) of the milk used to make the final product: cheese, yogurt, cottage cheese, etc.[6]

To explain further, nonfat milk has 80 calories in an eight-ounce carton. Zero percent of the calories comes from fat. An eight-ounce serving of "2% milk" has 130 calories and five grams of fat. The fat contributes 45 calories, or 35 percent of the calories of the milk, much more than the 2 percent that many people assume from the label. That places "2% milk" at a fat level higher than many of the leaner meat products. For instance, skinless chicken breast derives about 23 percent of its calories from fat. Whole milk is labeled as 5 percent fat, meaning that 5 percent of the weight of the milk comes from fat. Eight ounces of whole milk has 150 calories and derives about 48 percent of its calories from fat, roughly the same percent as lean steak.

The same comparisons can be made for all dairy products. A typical 1.5-ounce slice of cheddar has 160 calories. A low-fat slice has 120 calories, and a nonfat slice 60. That low-fat slice of cheddar has a label on it indicating it is low fat or made with low-fat (2%) milk; the consumer would be surprised to learn that 39 percent of the calories are from fat.

Food	Calories	Fat (g)	Calories from fat	% of calories from fat
Milk, 8-ounce serving				
Nonfat	80	0	0	0
Low fat (2%)	130	5	45	35
Whole fat (5%)	150	8	67	48
Cheddar, 1.5 ounces				
Nonfat	60	0	0	0
Low fat	120	5.2	47	39
Whole milk	160	13	117	73

Other forms of dairy are worse for weight control. They concentrate milk into ever more calorically dense forms such as cheese, sour cream, and yogurt. The government's dietary recommendations state that 1.5 ounces of cheese is equivalent to one cup of milk, but 1.5 ounces of cheese (the size of a nine-volt battery) contains roughly 170 calories, while the low-fat version contains 120 calories. Look at the chart below and think about how long it would take you to eat each food and how full you would feel.

Protein-containing food	Weight (oz.)	Protein (g)	Calories	Same size as a...
Milk, low fat	8	8	100	8-ounce snack-sized yogurt
Cheddar cheese, low fat	1.5	10	120	9-volt battery
Cooked black beans	4	7	110	Standard light bulb
Sugar snap peas	9	6	105	Baseball

The easiest way to incorporate most forms of dairy in your diet is as a flavoring and not as a substantial part of the meal. If you want a larger volume of dairy, consider yogurt—but be a discerning consumer. Most yogurts are loaded with added sugars and contain few or no live cultures, the beneficial bacteria that contribute to good intestinal health. Try plain, whole milk, non-homogenized yogurt, and scoop off the top layer of fat.

Why not eat regular, homogenized, low- or nonfat yogurt? That works, but non-homogenized[7] yogurt has a uniquely wholesome taste (the homogenization process alters the flavor). You can make a great low-calorie dessert with yogurt by mixing in fruit and a touch of non-caloric sweetener. Substituting yogurt-based salad dressings for oil-based dressings is another great way to cut calories while maximizing flavor. For more complex tastes for desserts and dressings experiment with additional ingredients: lemon juice, lime juice, cinnamon, vanilla, orange, and other natural flavor extracts.

In the last few years the dairy industry has made improvements in the flavor of many reduced-fat offerings: cheese, yogurt, sour cream, cream cheese, and cottage cheese. The progress in flavor comes from innovations in the use of fat-mimicking plant products: seaweed extracts (agar-agar, carrageenan, and alginates) and vegetable gums (xantham gum, locust bean, guar gum). These fat substitutes are considered safe, though a few alternative health practitioners believe that some, in particular carrageenan, can contribute to digestive problems. For many, the lower-fat dairy options have proven to be a critical part of a weight loss plan, but if you have a sensitive stomach it is worthwhile to experiment with eliminating fat substitutes from the diet.

Many weight loss clients report after a few weeks of using nonfat cottage cheese that they find it just as good as the full-fat version.

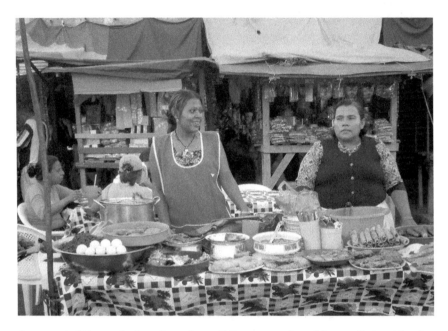

An upscale fritanga in downtown Leon. Fritangas — where Nicas sell street food — base their price solely on the protein. If you choose beans, your meal costs about $1. With chicken the price is over $2, and with beef, close to $3. The typical sides (cabbage salad, rice, fried plantains) have no effect on the price; you can take or leave them or even double them and the price won't budge. *It's all about the protein.*

NOTES

1 CDC. *National Health and Nutrition Examination Survey*, 2005-06.

2 Excess fat is that which goes beyond the essential fat needed for metabolic function, components of, and cushioning for organs. Protein guidelines assume a typical healthy range of body fat as 6 to 25% for men, 14 to 31% for women. Women who are below 21% fat and men below 14% fat are considered athletic body types. Under 14% for women and under 6% for men is considered problematic for health and can be indicative of eating disorders, malnutrition, or other disease states. When patients are overweight, dietitians do not use their actual weight to calculate protein needs. Instead, they calculate protein needs based on a formula called Ideal Body Weight.

   - For men: IBW = 106 pounds for the first 5 feet plus 6 pounds for each inch over 5 feet.
   - For women: IBW = 100 pounds for the 5 five feet plus 5 pounds for each inch over 5 feet.

   E.g., a 200-pound, 5'8" man does not need 72g of protein (0.36 × 200), he needs 55.5g (0.36 × 154).

3 While most of the body's tissues run on a flexible mix of fuels, the brain, nervous system, and red blood cells aren't flexible: they need a minimum of 130 grams of glucose per day. Since fat can't be converted into glucose, a low-carbohydrate diet forces the liver to convert proteins (from our muscles) into glucose. For this reason athletes are advised to eat sufficient carbohydrates—they are "protein sparing."

4 Colin Campbell, *The China Study* (Dallas, Texas: BenBella Books, 2006), 7.

5 Marion Nestle and Malden Nesheim, *Why Calories Count* (Oakland: University of California Press, 2012), 35.

6 There is innate variety in the industry. There are many breeds of cows, eating a large variety of feed, all of which impacts the composition of their milk. Some whole milk products are made with 5% fat milk, some with 4%. Techniques to reduce fat in milk are likewise variable. Some low-fat varieties use 2% milk, some 1.5%, others 1%; nonfat can range from 0% fat to 0.5%.

7 *Homogenization* slices up the fat particles in milk to make them much smaller. This prevents the fat from rising to the top and keeps it evenly dispersed in the milk. Homogenization occurs by passing milk under high pressure through a tiny opening. Some researchers believe in the controversial theory that the fat cells are reduced to such a small size that these cells can then enter into our arteries directly and cause heart disease. Whether that is true or not, it is true that homogenization creates novel shapes of fats that our bodies are not accustomed to encountering.

CHAPTER 8

The Sweet and the Fat

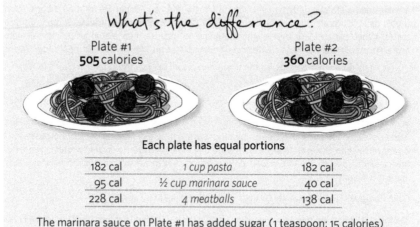

What's the difference?

Plate #1		Plate #2	
505 calories		**360** calories	

Each plate has equal portions

182 cal	*1 cup pasta*	182 cal
95 cal	*½ cup marinara sauce*	40 cal
228 cal	*4 meatballs*	138 cal

The marinara sauce on Plate #1 has added sugar (1 teaspoon: 15 calories) and oil (1 teaspoon: 40 calories), and the meatballs were made with beef that has a higher fat content, adding an extra 10 grams of fat (90 calories).

IN HIGH SCHOOL I WORKED FOR GREENPEACE. I knocked on strangers' doors in the hopes of raising awareness and money to tackle issues like the disappearing rainforest, aggressive Japanese whaling, and the increasing quantity of toxins in our water, air, and soil. As one unsuspecting resident after another learned a myriad of depressing facts—including firsthand knowledge of the distressing lack of grooming common to Greenpeace canvassers (me)—I learned an equally gloomy lesson. It was difficult to get people to care about faraway plants and animals and all the microscopic chemicals that might eventually accumulate in our tissues and cause us harm.

From the perspective of the dieter, fats and sweets have something in common with pollutants. When we look at two identical-appearing plates of food we can't easily determine differences in fat and sugar, nor can we can know which one is organic and which one is not. In the future, à la Mr. Spock from Star Trek, maybe we'll wave a sensor (or our smartphones) over our meals and a dietitian app will reveal all the components and how they relate to our health. That same concept would let us scan a picturesque landscape, our Greenpeace app revealing which pollutants lie hidden in the land, air, and water. Until that technology arrives we have to be aware that, whether in our food or in our environment, we often discount the impact of that which cannot be easily seen and measured.

This chapter puts this slippery subject under the microscope in order to assess the perils of—as well as the best options for—sweets and fats.

Diamonds in the Rough(age)

Sugar production is a refining process. The complex structure of plants like sugarcane, beets, and corn is broken down, and sugar is what's left over. Similarly, most of the fats we eat (butter, oil, and margarine) are in a highly concentrated form. Dissolution of the structural integrity of the source materials leaves behind purified calories so condensed that they are beyond structureless; they are nearly invisible.

In addition to invisibility, fats and sweets share other superhero (albeit in the dietary context, supervillain) powers.

Super energy: They are the nuclear energy of calories, densely packed, and taking up little volume.

Charisma: As any chef or food industry executive knows, almost every food is made far more enticing with the addition of fat, sugar, or both. A bonus is that both are cheap: if you're cutting corners (using ingredients that are less than fresh or of lower quality, rushing the cooking, serving small portions, etc.) you can cover up shortcomings with ease.

Unlike sugar, fat does not have inherently unhealthy qualities. The problem is that its caloric contribution is often wildly underestimated. This miscalculation can create a substantial drag on weight loss momentum. Fortunately, through fresher foods, herbs, spices, marinades, and other tricks of the culinary trade we can **lower our fat intake** without sacrificing much flavor. Likewise, we can **reduce our use of sweets** by being more aware of the sources and considering the judicious use of alternative sweeteners.

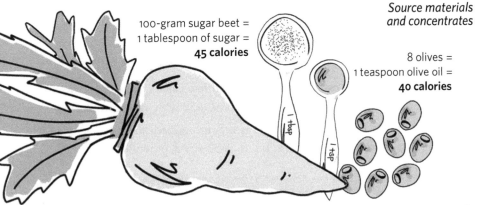

Source materials and concentrates

100-gram sugar beet =
1 tablespoon of sugar =
45 calories

8 olives =
1 teaspoon olive oil =
40 calories

Sweeteners: Calories, Chemicals, and Desire

Sweeteners can be divided into caloric and non-caloric types, and placed along a spectrum from less processed (found in a similar form in nature) to highly processed (significantly refined from source material) and artificial (synthesized in laboratories).

The most widely-consumed **caloric sweeteners** are refined from sugarcane, beets, and corn. These include white sugar, corn syrup and high-fructose corn syrup, and commercial sugar products used in processed foods (dextrose, fructose, maltose, maltodextrin, etc.). Less processed options include brown sugar and molasses and sugars derived from other sources: date sugar, maple syrup, coconut sugar, honey, sorghum syrup, and barley malt syrup.

- Many people are enticed by what they presume are the health benefits of less-processed sweeteners. They do taste great and contain some nutrients, but they have the *same weight-promoting effect as refined sweeteners.*

- All calorie-containing sweeteners fall under the broad nutritional definition of sugars. They are the simplest of carbohydrates: they're calorie dense, are digested rapidly, and don't satisfy appetite.

The most common **artificial, calorie-free sweeteners** in the U.S. are sucralose (Splenda*), aspartame (NutraSweet and Equal) and saccharin (Sweet 'n' Low).

- *The good news:* Many dieters feel "saved" by having low-calorie alternatives to their favorite desserts and drinks—they clearly can aid the transition to a lower-calorie diet. Their use appears especially effective in the first few weeks or months of the battle against the bulge and the sweet tooth.

- *The not-so-good news:* Although these artificial sweeteners are on the FDA's GRAS (Generally Recognized As Safe) list, there are also valid arguments against their long-term use. There are well-regarded studies[1] and many anecdotal reports linking their use to headaches, digestive problems, and, possibly, irregularities in blood sugar function. Because there is significant variation in the way humans process chemicals, this is a difficult area in which to get scientific consensus. These chemicals could have adverse effects on a minority of people while having no impact on the majority.

There are a handful of **natural calorie-free and low-calorie sweeteners** that, because of their more wholesome origins, can be used with more confidence.

- **Stevia** (Truvia, Pure Via, Sweetleaf) is a South American herb that has been used for thousands of years. It's available dried, or refined into liquid

---

* Sucralose is calorie free, but Splenda contains one gram of caloric sweetener (dextrose and maltodextrin) per packet. Splenda has about four calories per packet.

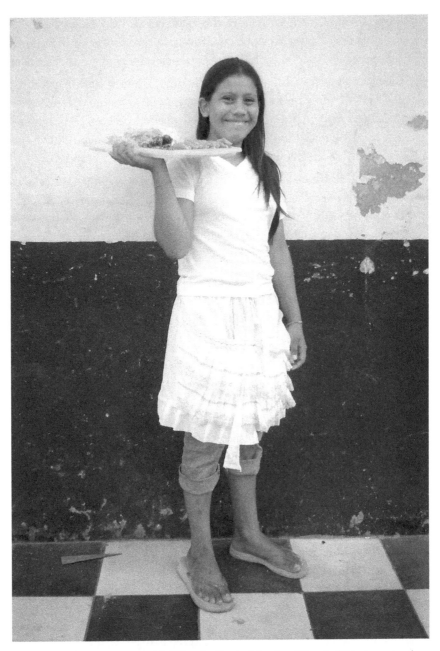

As Homer Simpson once said, "You don't win friends with salad." In Leon, twelve-year-old Lucretia sells homemade coconut caramels made out of finely shredded coconut, sugar, and food coloring. She is hoping to earn enough money to buy a uniform and books so that she can go to school.

Combining refined fat and sugar is a classic culinary strategy for maximizing plea-sure and creating profit. Would Lucretia do as well selling unrefined foods like carrot sticks or corn on the cob?

extracts and powders to remove the "plant" taste. It's also easy to grow. Fresh or dried leaves work best to sweeten drinks; some of the refined versions can be used in cooking. Stevia has no calories and is inexpensive.

- **Lohan, or monk fruit,** is an exceptionally sweet Chinese fruit that is dried and ground into a powder. You'll see lohan spelled several different ways (*luo han, lo han*); brands include Pure Monk and LoSweet. Delicious and nearly calorie free, its only downside is that it is one of the most expensive sweeteners on the market.

- **Xylitol** and **erythritol** are sugar alcohols.* Xylitol has about half the calories of common sweeteners, tastes great, and is priced between stevia and lohan. Erythritol (slightly pricier), also sold under the brand name Zero, has no calories. It has a slight cooling effect in the mouth, so it works better with cool-temperature foods than those meant to be eaten warm or hot.

These four options don't have to be used exclusively—you can mix and match them with other sweeteners. I like to combine a teaspoon of honey with a few drops of stevia extract when I sweeten yogurt, oatmeal, or tea.

It is important to keep in mind that *all types of sweeteners, regardless of composition or origin, signal the brain to increase the appetite.* That message is, essentially, "here is a safe, calorie-dense food, and you should eat a lot of it." Given the implications for weight gain I recommend reducing your sweetener consumption. This is particularly important for youth. Those whose early eating habits include frequent sweetener use will develop the expectation that food has to have a strong, sweet flavor to be enjoyable. Impressions made in youth are difficult to erase later in life.

It's Not Just Weight

If you haven't yet put down your honey nut muffin and backed slowly away, consider that caloric sweeteners affect more than just weight. They are mildly addictive and can contribute to fluctuations in energy, blood sugar, and mood. They also contribute to aging via the production of **advanced glycation end products**, the appropriately abbreviated AGEs. When you spill a sugary drink it sticks to everything. Sugar is also sticky on a molecular level. Excess sugar molecules can cause the protein molecules that compose our cells to

---

* **Sugar alcohols** include maltitol, maltitol syrup, sorbitol, mannitol, xylitol, lactitol, erythritol, and isomalt. Though they occur naturally in plants, the sugar alcohols we find in processed products are manufactured from sugars and starches. They are lower in calories than other sugars because the intestines cannot break them down completely. Unfortunately, this also means that using more than a modest amount can result in gas, bloating, and diarrhea. Xylitol and erythritol are the best tasting and easiest on the digestive system.

stick together (this process is called glycation) and cross-link. Cross-linked proteins can't fulfill their cellular obligations as efficiently. When enough cross-linked molecules accumulate in an organ (kidneys, lungs, arteries, brain), the decrease in function can contribute to the progression of many conditions, including kidney disease, diabetes, cardiovascular disease, and Alzheimer's. What's more, glycation makes skin less elastic and wrinkles deeper.

But I Just Can't Quit Cold Turkey...

As a recovering sugar junkie I assure you that there is hope. Fortunately, our taste buds have the memory of an indicted politician on trial. As your diet improves you'll notice a gradual reduction in the urgency of your sweet tooth. The less frequently you use sweeteners of any type, the more pronounced this effect will be.

While the ideal sweet is fruit, dieters who crave more excitement have many options. It's possible to modestly indulge your sweet tooth using one of two strategies. Neither has a definitive advantage for weight loss; choose the one that works for you:

The **natural strategy**: Eat typical desserts (ice cream, brownies, cookies), but in small portions or only as an occasional treat. The benefit is that you get the complete hedonistic experience that full fat and real sweeteners offer.

The **substitution strategy**: Food science offers us a tremendous variety of lower-calorie sweets. On the extremely low-calorie end of the spectrum are sugar- and fat-free jello and pudding. Slightly more caloric, and quite a bit more satisfying, are reduced-calorie frozen desserts. Quality brands include Arctic Zero, Enlightened, Halo Top, and Skinny Cow. There are also many varieties of low-calorie frozen yogurt. The benefit of substitution is that portions can be "normal-sized" and you don't have to reserve indulgences for special occasions.

Hidden Sugars

Sweet treats are the logical first place to start when cutting down on sugar, but you'll also find that **sugar is widely dispersed in processed food.** It's often lurking in the list of ingredients under one of its various pseudonyms: maltose, dextrose, etc. It's added to condiments and sauces, frozen entrées, cereal, french fries, canned vegetables and fruits, baked beans, processed and deli meats, soup, jam, salad dressing, peanut butter, and many more items.

Pay attention to labels. Spend a few extra moments in the grocery aisle and you can usually find a low-sugar or sugar-free alternative to your favorite brand.

Taste is all about comparative experiences. Your enjoyment of reduced-calorie treats is proportional to how long ago you ate conventional treats. In other words, if you rarely have sweets, an Arctic Zero dessert will taste terrific. If you ate a traditional ice cream sundae yesterday, Arctic Zero won't taste nearly as good. The more distant the sweet, full-calorie desserts are in your memory, the more satisfaction you'll get from lower-calorie options. Fortunately, the sweet-tastes-increase-desire cycle works perfectly well in reverse. With a little patience, you may eventually find the sweet taste of fresh fruit to be all you need.

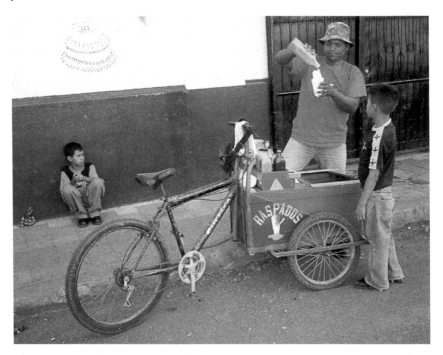

Those mamoncillo never had a chance. Esteban sells *raspados*, shaved ice topped with either condensed milk or a fruit syrup, both of which are highly sweetened. Esteban, like many Nicaraguans, has no idea that sugar is bad for you. In fact, like people in many developing nations, few Nicaraguans have the scientific literacy to make a strong connection between the diet they eat and their health. Note the unregarded branch of *mamoncillo* fruit next to the seated boy. Mamoncillo is tangy and sweet, grows all over Nicaragua, and costs a few pennies for a branch of 20 to 30 fruits. (*Leon*)

Raspados, *carmelos*, and a large variety of other sweets and beverages contribute to Nicaragua's annual per capita rate of sugar consumption of more than 100 pounds (more than half a cup per day), or about 15 percent of the diet. Sugar wasn't always so common. The first sugar factory in Nicaragua didn't open until 1892, and consumption remained low until a few generations ago.[2]

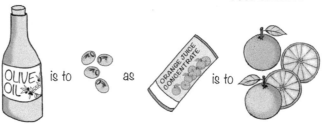

Fats

As with sweeteners, the availability and purity of fats have grown rapidly in recent generations. Pure fats like oil and butter are relatively new to the human diet, appearing shortly after the advent of agriculture. At first they were rare; producing them was resource intensive and difficult, and the products were perishable. What were our fat sources before purified fats became common?

People in the tropics, including parts of Nicaragua, sometimes cooked with coconut oil. Women mashed up coconut to make coconut milk. They let it sit until the oil rose to the top, after which they separated and collected it using the heat from a candle or small cook fire. The process was time consuming and produced only a small of amount of oil with a short shelf life. The constraints of home production promoted modest use. Fortunately, the rich flavor of the fresh oil meant that a few teaspoons were sufficient to sauté fish and vegetables.

In many other regions of the world, villages had community presses with which to make fresh oils from local sources like sesame, flax, or olives. Unprocessed oils imbued traditional dishes with weighty, pungent flavors.

Animal fat was also used: whenever animals were slaughtered, their fat was collected and rendered. (**Rendering**, used in the processing of both wild and livestock animals, separates edible fats from protein and other materials.) Like fresh vegetable oils, animal fats have vibrant flavor and a short shelf life.

In the 20th century new methods of oil production and farming allowed for a significant drop in the cost of bottled vegetable oils. By the mid-20th century the industrialized West's use of processed oils surpassed its use of traditional fats. In recent decades the developing world has also seen steadily rising consumption of processed oil.

The increase could be due to the convenience of buying bottled oil, though another subtle factor may be the lack of flavor in modern oil. One needs to use more processed oil to satisfy the taste buds.

....

Manipulating the Market: In the 1950s, large commercial vegetable oil companies came to Nicaragua and ran ad campaigns to persuade the public to switch to their cheap, shelf-stable bottled oil. Their ads associated poor people in traditional dress and homes with the use of homemade coconut oil, while vegetable-oil consumers were modern, wealthy, and well dressed. (Read more about marketing and influence in **Chapter 12.**)

Why is it that modern oils lack "personality"?

Oils are extracted from whole foods (seeds, nuts, and grains) by removing the protein, carbohydrate, fiber, and water to isolate the fat. This process parallels the refining of sugarcane, corn, and beets into sweeteners. In all cases the manufacturing process can be quite complex, depending on the source material and the specific sweetener or oil produced. In the case of oil production, the processing chain can include any or all of these: chemical solvents (most often hexane, a petroleum product), high heat, high pressure, and bleaching. A final treatment can include chemical preservatives to prolong shelf life and deodorizing agents to disguise the rancid-smelling byproducts of the refining process. Most of the nutritious components of the oils (lecithin, vitamins, minerals, chlorophyll, and phospholipids) are removed or destroyed.[3] The delicate molecules that give oil its distinct character and flavor disappear alongside the other micronutrients. Consumers' concerns about these practices, along with their desire for better-tasting oils, have fueled a market for less-processed oils. However, *even the finest quality, freshest, extra-virgin, cold-pressed oil is still a highly-processed food.*

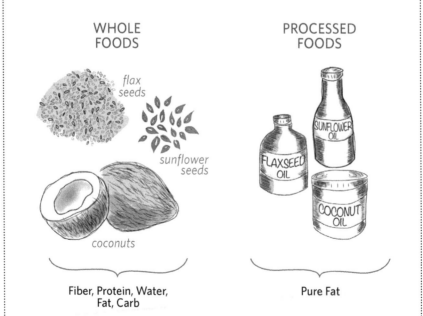

WHOLE
FOODS

PROCESSED
FOODS

flax seeds

sunflower seeds

coconuts

Fiber, Protein, Water,
Fat, Carb

Pure Fat

Get the Most Flavor From Your Fat

The use of vegetable oil is a compromise when you're emphasizing whole foods in your diet. If you do use oil, look for **cold-temperature, expeller-pressed** oils. These are extracted without chemical solvents and with lower heat and pressure. If the producers are conscientious about their techniques, the resulting oils should smell and taste like their source material. For example:

- Cold-pressed sesame oil will have a powerful sesame smell and taste. Less-expensive oil with no production information on the label will have a lighter flavor and a negligible smell.

- Note the difference between extra-virgin olive oil and oil labeled "pure olive oil" or just "olive oil." The extra-virgin designation (if the bottle is labeled honestly[4]) indicates that the oil comes from the first pressing. It will have a deep green color, provide a complex and inviting taste, and smell like olives. The other types of oil are made from second and third pressings. The heat and pressure used are higher, and the result is akin to making a photocopy of a photocopy: a lighter color, a significantly diminished olive flavor, and a fainter smell.

Use a small amount of **animal fat** (lard or chicken fat) or fatty meat, such as bacon, sausage, or beef, when you boil legumes or sauté your main dish of vegetables. A thumb-sized piece of meat is enough to give lentils, split peas, and beans a fuller and more enticing flavor. A smidgen of animal fat does the trick for vegetables as well. One of my favorite vegetables dishes is a head of cabbage sautéed with sea salt, caraway seeds, and a half-strip of bacon or half of a sausage. Another favorite is baked french fries made with a touch of lard—they give traditional fried french fries a run for the money.

Rather than using purified fats, use **foods that contain fat.** Naturally high-fat foods (cheese, yogurt, nuts and seeds, avocados, olives, and coconut) can be sprinkled into your dishes. Even small quantities add intense flavors. For example, instead of sautéing a piece of chicken in oil, bake it. Sprinkle it with parmesan cheese and slivered almonds. The calories from fat will be about the same as sautéing, but you will have made an improvement in both flavor and nutritional quality.

Instead of cooking with fat, **add fat at the table.** Cooking with fat only degrades its quality and flavor. Adding fat at the table (butter, oil, cheese, grated nuts, olives) delivers more compelling flavor and it makes it easier to track quantity and calories.

Saturated Fats = Heart Disease? Not necessarily. When you burn more calories than you consume there are no leftover fats to clog arteries.

Main course or side, we like it fried.

Most food in Nicaragua is fried. Bottled vegetable oil wasn't introduced to the country until the 1950s, but now accounts for approximately 15 percent of the calories in the country's daily diet.

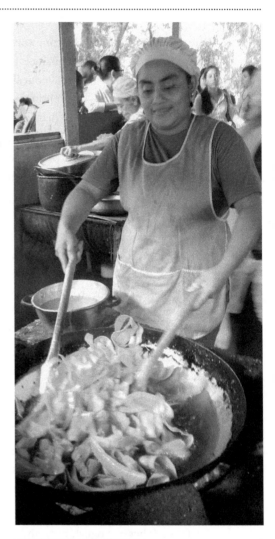

At the UNAN cafeteria in Managua, Lupita pulls out a fresh batch of *tajadas* (fried plantains) from a vat of boiling oil. Most students' lunches feature fried plantains and/or fried rice. A common dish is *tajadas con queso o carne*, a heaping pile of deep-fried plantains topped with three ounces of cheese or meat and a sprinkling of cabbage. Meals are always accompanied by a sweet beverage, most often Coke.

Considered Nicaragua's national dish, *gallo pinto* ("spotted rooster") is fried white rice and beans. Interestingly, most of the calories in gallo pinto come from vegetable oil and rice, two foods that weren't commonly consumed in Nicaragua until late in the 20th century. This begs the question: how quickly can a dish become a nation's iconic meal and how exactly does this happen?

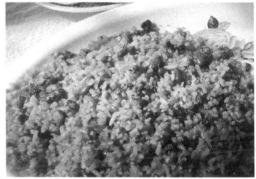

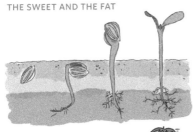

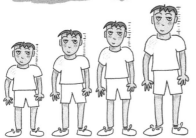

Nuts and Seeds: Proteins or Fats?

A seed begins its life cycle by falling to the ground and being covered by soil and debris. When spring arrives it anchors itself with roots and sends a shoot upwards to grow its first leaves. Until the plant can grow enough leaves to photosynthesize energy and grow deep enough roots to pull nutrients from the soil, it survives on the calorie-dense nutrient mix inside the seed.

Nuts and seeds, on average, derive nearly 75 percent of their calories from fat. The remainder is split between protein and carbohydrate. Oddly, some food systems classify nuts and seeds as proteins. I classify them as fats. Not surprisingly, they are ideal for those who are underweight or undergoing periods of growth or healing (pregnancy, puberty, recovering from surgery or illness). The rest of us should use nuts and seeds moderately, as a way to flavor meals in place of oil and butter.

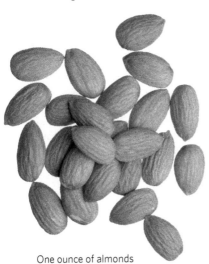

One ounce of almonds
is about 22 to 25 nuts.

Nuts and Seeds: A Closer Look

	Total Calories	Calories from...		
		Fat	Protein	Carb
Nuts				
Cashews	157	108	20	32
Peanuts	161	126	28	20
Almonds	164	126	24	24
Seeds				
Pumpkin	158	126	26	12
Hemp	160	126	36	10
Sunflower	164	126	24	24
Corn (7 oz.)	161	18	21	145

Compare corn kernels and cashews. Per calorie, corn has the same amount of protein.

All nuts and seeds are raw, one-ounce portions.
Serving size calculated without inedible shells/hulls.
Data comes from the USDA.

Did you notice? The numbers don't add up. Calories from carbohydrate include fiber. Some fiber — particularly insoluble fiber, in which nuts and seeds are high — passes through the body unabsorbed. The U.S. Food and Drug Administration allows food labels to subtract insoluble fiber calories from the total calories. This accounts for the total calories being a little less than the sum of the calories from the components.

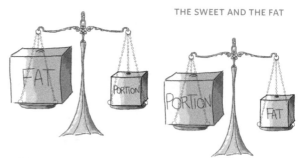

How Much Fat?

It's a matter of budgeting. There are many factors discussed in this book (immersion, activity, stress, sleep, a balanced plate, fiber, and food processing) that have impacts on the calorie budget. All things being equal, however, the debate on fat boils down to a choice between portion size and fat content. I've noticed that men often prefer sacrificing the fat for stomach-filling large portions, while women lean toward sacrificing portions and keeping the fat. Some people, particularly those who are working on vanity weight, do well with a diet moderate in fat (20 to 35 percent) or even high in fat (above 35 percent). For those with substantial weight to lose (more than 10 percent of their body weight) I see more success when fat calories drop below 20 percent.

During substantial weight loss the body responds in an unfortunately counterproductive way: an array of hormonal and metabolic responses increase appetite while slowing metabolism. (This contributes to the difficulty dieters have achieving long-term success.) When this happens your taste buds have an easier time adjusting to the flavor of less fat than your appetite has adjusting to smaller portions. In other words, the drive to eat for flavor is not as strong as the drive to eat from an insufficiently full stomach. Regardless of the amount of fat you use, be conscious of how much it is contributing to your caloric budget.

Vanity weight is non-medically related extra weight. It represents the modest amount of weight (less than 10% of total weight) you want to lose to look better in a bathing suit, for example, as opposed to the weight you need to lose to reduce your blood pressure or blood sugar.

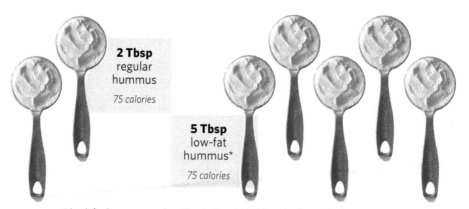

2 Tbsp
regular
hummus

75 calories

5 Tbsp
low-fat
hummus*

75 calories

* Look for hummus made without oil or tahini. See the **Appendix** for low-calorie options.

Watching fat intake is effective for five reasons:

1 Fats, at 9 calories per gram, have more than twice as many calories as carbohydrates and proteins, which both contain 4 calories per gram.

2 High-fat foods tend be low in water and fiber, reducing their capacity to fill you.

3 All excess calories are converted into fat. However, since dietary fats closely resemble human fat, the liver can convert dietary fat into body fat with remarkable efficiency. (See thermic effect, Chapter 4.) On average it takes 3 calories of energy to turn 100 calories of dietary fat into body fat. It takes 23 calories of energy to turn 100 calories of carbohydrate into body fat.[5]

4 High-fat meals can burden the liver, leaving us tired and nauseated. For this reason hospital patients with poor liver health are routinely put on low-fat diets to ease liver recovery.

5 This last reason is rarely discussed: Because fat carries flavor, decreasing its use in the diet performs a "dietary exorcism." The ability of food to overpower the senses, to induce cravings, is diminished when we lower our fat intake. For those of us who struggle with cravings and willpower, decreasing fat can be a powerful — if temporarily challenging — strategic move.

You can lower your fat intake by:

1 Reading labels and looking up the foods you eat most often to identify sources and quantities of fat in your diet

2 Avoiding pure fats (butter, oil, margarine) and exercising caution with naturally high-fat foods (dairy, high-fat meat or fish, nuts, seeds, olives, avocados, etc.)

3 Choosing low- or nonfat foods and avoiding typical high-fat processed foods (anything fried, most baked goods, all junk food, and fast food)

4 Being careful when you dine out. When you're ordering at a restaurant, ask that your meal be prepared without added fats such as butter and oil.

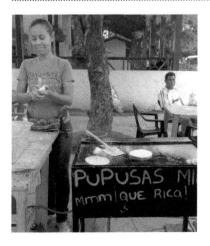

Mmm ¡Que Rica! When I talked to cooks in both Nicaragua and the U.S., a common comment was that *higher-fat dishes outsell lower-fat options.* People everywhere instinctively prefer the taste of calorie-dense foods. Cooks know this and are quick to use generous amounts of fat to prepare meals. Even options that sound healthy (salads, grilled meat or fish) are often loaded with subtle sources of fat: cheese, nuts, heavy dressings, and oil- and butter-based sauces and marinades. If you don't know how many calories are in a dish or are unaware of the health consequences of eating too many calories, it is unlikely that you will choose less calorically dense options. (*Managua*)

What About Traditional High-Fat Diets?

Weston Price and his devotee Sally Fallon wrote persuasively about the benefits of many traditional high-fat diets in *Nutrition and Physical Degeneration* and *Nourishing Traditions*. In the past decade many more health experts have jumped on the high-fat bandwagon. It is always a good marketing technique to tell people the "good news"—salvation is at hand and it will taste great: oil, butter, bacon, cheese, walnuts, and chocolate!

While it is true that the diets of many traditional cultures (particularly those in colder regions of the world) were high in fat, the lives of traditional peoples were quite different from the life of the average person seeking weight loss today. They were highly active, ate almost entirely whole-food diets with minimal or no food processing, and experienced periods of food scarcity (involuntary fasting brought on by weak harvests and/or scarce hunting). If we were to adopt their diets as a cure we would also have to adopt their lifestyles.

I don't crusade against fat indiscriminately; a whole-food, high-fat diet can be ideal for some people with no history of weight struggles. I've designed Price- and Fallon-inspired diets for patients who were either underweight or at a healthy body weight, and they have thrived. For those who desire significant weight loss, moderate-fat diets (20 to 35 percent of calories) and high-fat diets (more than 35 percent of calories) mean that success is only possible with either strict discipline in portion sizes or a dramatic increase in activity.

The Role of Fats in Medical Nutrition Therapy

USDA guidelines for healthy adults recommend that 20 to 35 percent of your daily intake of calories be from fat. However, in the same way that a low-fat diet (less than 20 percent of calories) can be an appropriate tool to aid weight loss, there are times when high-fat diets play a crucial role in health.

Dietitians prescribe high-fat diets in many situations, including:

- **Hospitalization:** Surgery, infections, illness, burns, and broken bones can cause temporary surges in calorie needs. If these needs aren't met, involuntary weight loss can result, which slows healing. High-fat diets meet those needs, prevent weight loss, and keep healing on track.

- **Loss of appetite** (often due to medication): Fat's appetite-stimulating properties help patients regain an interest in eating.

- **Women who are underweight while pregnant:** This often happens with teenage pregnancies and with women who experience significant morning sickness. A high-fat diet speeds weight gain and helps ensure a healthy baby and mother.

Uses of fat	Function	Replacement
Culinary	Flavor	Fresh(er) ingredients, herbs, spices, marinades
	Pan lubricant	Nonstick pans, sprays, nonfat cooking techniques
	Moisten food	Puréed fruit or vegetables
Biological	Warmth	A jacket, a sweater, long underwear
	Energy storage	A refrigerator, pantry, cupboards
	Cell walls, hormones, etc.	The liver can make all needed fats except for essential fatty acids (discussed in the following pages)

The Culinary and Biological Roles of Fats

Having covered all the reasons we might want to put down the butter knife, it's worth flipping the argument and looking at why we need fat. In the culinary realm fats serve three purposes: to provide and carry flavor, to lubricate the cooking vessel (pan, pot, etc.), and to moisten food. Fat is desirable because it adds its own inherent flavor, carries and intensifies the flavor components of other food, and has what culinary scientists call "mouthfeel" (alternatively described as texture and richness).

When a fat tastes bland (as do most bottled oils), people make up for it by increasing the quantity to amplify the mouthfeel. When you use more flavorful fats (see page 95) it takes less to satisfy your craving. You can further reduce your need to add fat for flavor by using fresh ingredients and being creative with low- and nonfat marinades, herbs, spices, broth, wine, and bouillon. Many cooking techniques work well without added fat. Try steaming, baking, poaching, stewing, and grilling. You can lower the need for lubrication by using nonstick pans and spray oils, which, because of their efficient dispersion process, make it easier to cook with less oil. When cooking and baking you can replace the moisture provided by fat with fruit and vegetable purées. Commercial fat replacers are available—Smuckers and Sunkist make two of the more popular products—and you can experiment with your own substitutions.

There are a handful of roles fat plays in the body, such as hormone synthesis and making up part of cell walls. Excess fat's biological functions are energy storage and warmth. Historically, extra fat was an internal refrigerator—a way to store calories for times when food was scarce, when hunts or harvests were unsuccessful. The warmth function is a little less universal; nevertheless, in colder climates and seasons extra fat did keep our internal organs warm and protected. These historical roles for fat have been replaced in modern times by clothing, refrigerators, and shelf-stable foods.

Low-Fat Diets and Essential Fatty Acids

Is there danger in diets that drop below 20 percent fat? The answers are yes, no, and maybe. There are three points to consider:

1 **Fat needs differ** for those at a healthy body weight and those who are overweight. If you're slim it's possible to develop a deficiency; you shouldn't try low-fat. If you're overweight you're carrying extra fat, and if your diet isn't providing enough fat your body will pull fat (including essential fatty acids) from your own tissues. In other words, it's difficult to develop a dietary deficiency of a nutrient that your body contains in excess.

2 **Humans can thrive on a wide range of diets.** Many traditional diets, particularly in tropical zones, are low in fat. The year-round growing season and moderate temperatures mean that excess body fat isn't needed as calorie storage or insulation. Unsurprisingly, the people—and the animals they eat—tend to have low body fat. Dietary surveys show that traditional tropical diets are typically composed of 60 to 80 percent carbohydrates, 10 to 15 percent protein and 15 to 20 percent fat. Some traditional diets contain only 10 percent fat.[6]

3 Even on a very low-fat diet **the body rarely goes into deficiency** because the liver can manufacture nearly all the fats we need from any source—carbohydrates, proteins, or fats.

There are only two exceptions to the liver's fat-production capabilities: omega-3 and omega-6 fatty acids. For this reason they are classified as **essential fatty acids** (EFAs). The most common culinary oils are the highest in omega-6: soy, corn, safflower, cottonseed, and peanut. Because these oils are heavily used in food processing the Western diet has the highest intake of omega-6 fatty acids in the world and deficiencies are exceptionally rare. Omega-3 fatty acids, on the other hand, are less common in our modern diet.

Preindustrial diets had a close-to-even ratio of omega-3 to omega-6, while the average American diet is estimated to have about 10 to 20 times more omega-6 than omega-3. Because of EFAs' multiple roles in maintaining health, a skewed ratio exacerbates inflammation-related conditions such as heart disease, some cancers, Alzheimer's, arthritis, and obesity. Physicians routinely prescribe omega-3 fatty acid supplements for these conditions. However, the same effect—the restoration of the omega equilibrium—could be achieved by lowering omega-6 intake. Of course, physicians know compliance is better when patients are simply asked to pop some pills rather than make dramatic changes in their diets.

Though it is uncommon to have a deficit of omega-3 fatty acids in your diet, it's important to know the consequences of a deficiency.

Short-term deficiency can result in dry hair and/or skin, while long-term deficiency contributes to heart disease, depression, poor circulation, and weakened immunity.

If a deficiency is suspected, you have **options**.

	portion	omega-3	total fat
wild salmon	4 oz.	2g	10g
walnuts	¼ cup	2g	16g

- *Food sources:* Some fish and nuts are high in omega-3 fatty acids, but it is usually a small percentage of the total fat content. If you're trying to lose weight, a supplement might be a better choice. Two foods with the highest omega-3 content are wild salmon (20 percent) and walnuts (14 percent).

- *Dietary supplements:* Take 3-10 grams of an omega-3 supplement daily. Check with your dietitian or physician to confirm precise dosage and to check if the supplement will interact with your medications.

The ratio shift is partly due to the worldwide increase in commercial oil use in the diet, and partly due to a revolution in agricultural processes. Domesticated animals were traditionally grazed on pasture, which provides omega-3 fatty acids. Starting in the 1930s, farmers began to favor corn and soy feed, which allowed them to move animals from free-range grazing to concentrated feedlots. Grains and legumes are far more calorie dense than foliage, so the animals gained weight at a blistering pace, and profits increased proportionally. Given the economics, it was only a few decades before almost all livestock animals went from a "sober plate" (nutritionally balanced, with a near-even ratio of EFAs) to a "heavy plate" (higher in calories, with more omega-6 than omega-3).

The parallels between the animal and the human worlds are hard to ignore. As our lives have become more sedentary, so have the lives of the animals we eat. As those animals began to forgo lighter plant materials (greens and foliage) for denser sources of calories (starches and proteins), so did we; we all gained weight (and skewed our EFA ratios). In recent years there has been a return to raising animals on pasture, as consumers are willing to pay a premium for healthier animal products. Ironically, we are paying extra for animals to eat light, healthy diets though we are often hesitant to do the same.

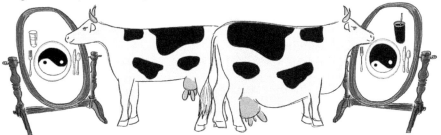

The Food Sobriety diet is a heavily plant-based diet that reduces processed fats. Your ratio of omega-3 to omega-6 fatty acids will improve even if your total fat intake falls.

Saturated and Unsaturated Fats

One of the qualities that makes healthy fats like omega-3 fatty acids beneficial is that they are **unsaturated**. Their molecular structure is characterized by double carbon bonds, which form irregular (kinked or curved) shapes that can't stack together tightly or form solids easily; they interact like potato chips in a bag. **Saturated** fats only have single carbon bonds, which gives them a straight shape and allows them to stack together like sticks of gum in a pack. This spatial arrangement is the reason saturated fats remain solid at room temperatures. In your body saturated fats can stick together and make cells less flexible, or form blockages, which in blood vessels can slow circulation and eventually lead to cardiovascular disease.

The adage sounds simple: unsaturated fats are better than saturated ones, right? Unfortunately, it's a touch more complex. The "unhealthy" saturated fats are stable and can take heat, pressure, and light with minimal damage. The "healthy" unsaturated oils that are abundant in many plant foods, including nuts, seeds, and vegetable oils, cannot. Double bonds are highly reactive, and with heat, light, or pressure, they become damaged via free radical oxidation. As mentioned before, in preindustrial times oils made from unsaturated foods were made in small batches with minimal heat and pressure, so the oils stayed fresh until used.

Today, the same foods that are acclaimed for their "healthy fat" content are likely to have many of those healthy qualities degraded long before the product reaches your grocery cart. *If you want the benefits of healthy fats and you have the calories to spare in your dietary budget, stick to unprocessed natural fats in their original "packaging."* Skip the olive oil, almond butter, and coconut oil. Instead eat olives, almonds, and coconuts. Ideally, buy nuts and seeds unshelled; the shell preserves the delicate unsaturated fats.

NOTES

1 Jotham Suez et al. "Artificial sweeteners induce glucose intolerance by altering the gut microbiota." Nature 514 (2014), 1476-4687.

2 Paul Hoebink, *Sugar from Nicaragua* (Nijmegen, Netherlands: Centre for International Development Issues Nijmegen, Radboud University, June 2014), 16. PDF.

3 Udo Erasmus, *Fats That Heal, Fats That Kill: The Complete Guide to Fats, Oils, Cholesterol and Human Health* (Tennessee: Alive Books, 1993), 85-89.

4 Cecilia Rodriguez. "The Olive Oil Scam: If 80% Is Fake, Why Do You Keep Buying It?" *Forbes.com*, Feb. 10, 2016.

5 Daniel S. Kirshenbaum, *The Healthy Obsession Program: Smart Weight Loss Instead of Low-Carb Lunacy* (Dallas: BenBella Books, 2005), 107.

6 Darna L. Dufour, "Diet and nutritional status of Amerindians: a review of the literature." *Cadernos de Saúde Pública* 7 (1991), 481-502.

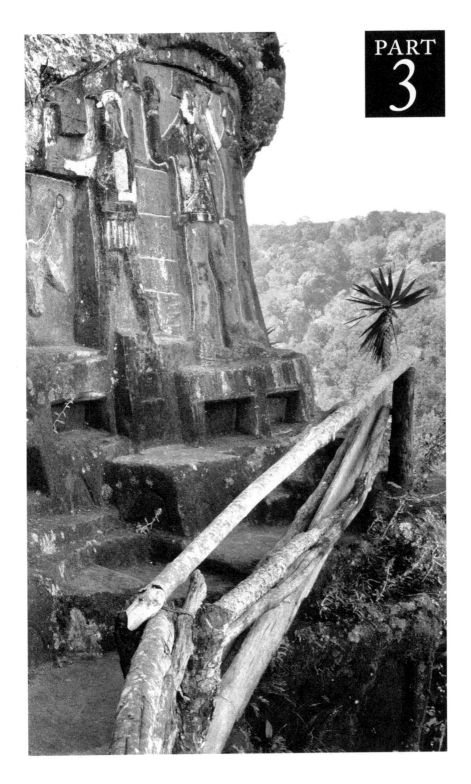

CHAPTER 9

Romancing the Plate

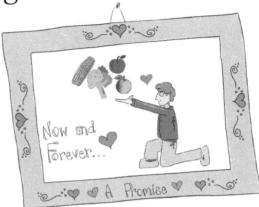

OUR IDENTITY IS SHAPED BY OUR RELATIONSHIPS with family, friends, co-workers, and romantic partners. What do we give and receive? Is there balance? We invest time and energy (grief, money, blood, sweat, and tears...) in relationships because we hope they'll improve our lives.

Developing a positive relationship with food deserves a similar degree of time and attention because the right diet will significantly improve our lives. This chapter focuses on two aspects of our dietary relationships: expectations and immersion.

Expectations: Creating a Realistic Perspective on Diet

Just a Fling or the Real Thing?

An indulgent diet is like an affair with a married partner—he or she might be gorgeous, hilarious, and generous, but won't acknowledge you in public. The fantasy of a more meaningful relationship is wonderful, but the reality is fleeting pleasures eclipsed by long periods of loneliness. To compound the metaphor: eating rich and sweet food is like a one-night stand. You might well anticipate the thrill, but satisfaction is fleeting while regret lingers.

You're not going to choose a lifelong partner from the guys catcalling you on the corner or those last drunken revelers in the bar. Nor do you want to build a long-term relationship with pasta Alfredo and meatballs. Judge a diet for its potential. Where will it take you in one, five, or even ten years? *Eating for instant gratification is the ultimate short-term relationship. It is a fear of commitment to self.*

Did you lose your appetite when you read about my budget diet in Nicaragua? Likely so, but that diet, despite my initial struggles, brought me enduring health. Does anyone look back on rich meals eaten and think, "Thank god I ate that?" To this day, every time I see beans, corn, or vegetables I smile in appreciation. Given time you will develop gratitude for any diet that makes you light and energetic.

Don't waste your time with flirtatious partners. Unlike our other relationships, the one
with food is capable of rapid transformation
because we are the only sentient part of the
couple. No matter how much it seems that
ice cream is calling out your name, it won't cry
in your absence. And when you call it quits
with protein bars and sports drinks they won't
come sprinting after you, drunkenly text you,
or write you long, weepy emails.

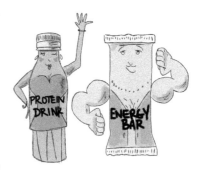

All We Want Is Perfection — Is That So Wrong?

Burgers with sunset yellow-orange cheese slices, gently ruffled lettuce, and perfectly formed rolls with an artistic scattering of sesame seeds. Rainbow-colored breakfast cereals with layered sugar crystals and artful splashes of milk. Golden brown, flaky-crust pies filled with bright red, flawlessly round cherries and cut in geometrically precise wedges. Steaming racks of ribs gleaming with barbeque sauce. Ice-cold beer in a curvy, frosty glass. Like art, commercial images of food have power. These images are the modern-day versions of the Sistine Chapel, leaving us spellbound by the glorious abundance: an overstimulating blend of rich colors and large portions, replete with sweet, dense calories.

The food industry has become a priesthood devoted to the manufacture and promotion of these meticulous idealized standards, heavenly food fantasies that demand our worship. This priesthood even has a unique niche profession, Michelangelos of food dedicated to perfecting the images. Food stylists are highly trained artists who use paint, plastic models, makeup, glue, glycerin, and oils to make the mundane look magnificent.

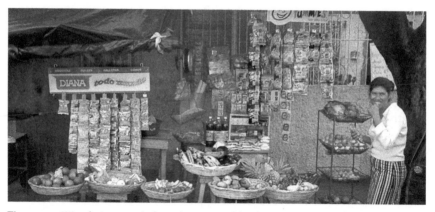

The competition between whole and processed foods is on display at most road stands in Nicaragua. Like people everywhere, Nicas are attracted to the exciting flavors, colors, and textures of calorie-dense processed foods. Not realizing that processed foods are less nutritious, many assume the opposite: that anything processed, packaged, and imported is superior to anything local and unprocessed. *(Managua)*

The unrealistic pictures of the food we eat parallel the way we promote unrealistic ideals for the body. Women have long objected to the fact that images of women in the media set impossibly high standards for beauty. To obtain and maintain the right looks, models and celebrities often rely on diet pills, cosmetic surgery, grueling exercise regimens and extreme diets, cleanses, and fasts. Photographs are routinely altered to make subjects look thinner, eliminate real or perceived imperfections, and exaggerate positive features. Men no longer escape this pressure—images of men regularly feature six-pack abs, bulging muscles, and chiseled movie-star faces. For both our bodies and our diets, we are increasingly conditioned to expect perfection.

The media and the fashion/beauty industry are rightly criticized for promoting unrealistic body image, yet the sky-high expectations and desires the food industry creates somehow escape critique. At the intersection of desire and appetite you'll find the image-makers, catering to an ever-escalating cycle of aspiration. Their pitch: Not everyone can embody the most desirable traits or have a scintillating romantic partner, but we can all eat highly flavorful foods. *("Try Ben & Jerry's Bonnaroo Buzz: 'Light coffee & malt ice cream with whiskey caramel swirls & English toffee pieces'!")* The hoped-for takeaway: If you can't make it out to the festival and create your own ecstatic dance party, at least you can have a taste of equivalent joy.

In the 1950s and '60s, when processed foods were still fairly new to the market, you could count on one hand the number of ice cream flavors for sale. With each passing year the number of flavors increased. Many foods that originally had no added flavor (like nuts, coffee creamer, beef jerky, and potato chips) are now available in astonishing variety.

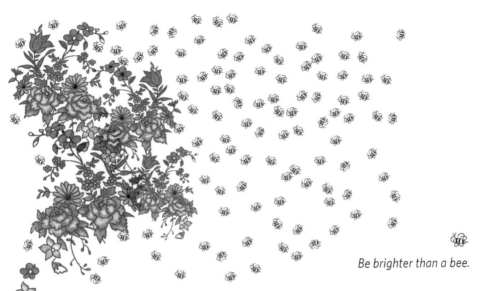

Be brighter than a bee.

Imagine that the food industry is a field of flowers and the customers are a swarm of bees. Just as flowers compete to attract more pollinators (*their* customers) by offering bright colors, sweet nectar, appealing fragrances, and a variety of petal shapes, the food industry offers vibrant packaging, "new-and-improved" features, wild flavor combinations, and synthetic shortcuts (artificial flavors, scents, and colors). The foodie movement is engaged in the same arms race as the rest of the processed-food industry, although the gains are via a more organic method: complex, often calorie-dense recipes that skip the synthetics in favor of fresh ingredients chosen for their inherent flavor, not low cost. Whether it's Cool Ranch Doritos or Kool Ranch kale chips, the 21st-century, Willy Wonka-fied food landscape makes it a challenge to build an appetite for simple, natural foods.

Pornography Is Pornography Is Pornography

Our ever-escalating expectations are the intended consequence of a powerful marketing technique called "food porn." Although it is unclear just who first defined the term, one of the early usages was in Frederick Kaufman's 2005 *Harper's* article "Debbie Does Salad: The Food Network at the Frontiers of Pornography."[1] The article revealed how the photographers and cameramen of the food industry adopted the visual techniques that pornographers developed.

The link goes further: in *The Brain That Changes Itself*, Dr. Norman Doidge studied the relationship between pornography and sexual arousal.[2] He concluded that images of attractive and submissive women conditioned male viewers to the point that they had difficulty becoming aroused by normal women in conventional settings. Increased exposure resulted in the subjects being less aroused by both their actual partners and their virtual ones. The subjects demonstrated classic patterns of addiction, with increasing time committed to the habit and a desire for ever-stronger imagery.

As with sex, we have taken the wholesome, natural act of eating and redefined it. At first it was the food industry that raised the bar with more seductive food and the accompanying explicit marketing. Now society en masse has picked up the baton and is in engaged in a 'round-the-clock, social-media-fueled, food-beauty pageant marathon.

Dr. Doidge's treatment for porn addiction was surprisingly simple. With a slow, steady reduction in viewing most patients were able to give up their habit entirely and regain a normal level of interest in and contentment with their sexual partners. The same process occurs with food. As your exposure to all forms of media food fetish (Instagram, Pinterest, Facebook, magazines, TV, etc.) decreases, your expectations will normalize and your satisfaction with all food will increase. Exposure—either its presence or absence—is a primary driver of behavior. Similarly, the longer you consume the Food Sobriety diet, the more your taste buds adapt.

Your Life On Display

What's more important—your date or letting your friends and followers know about your date? What about your meals? Are you focused on eating to maintain your health, or are you making sure you publicize your daring taste, ability to score a coveted reservation, and fabulous social life?

When you post photos of your gourmet dining experiences, your vacation, or your relationship highlights, be conscious of what you're trying to do. Are you just keeping in touch? Showing off? Desperately trying to maintain the illusion that everything is perfect? Most of us carefully curate our profiles to show an ideal vision of ourselves to the public. When this is aspirational, it can be (mostly) harmless. When you're using it to create a fantasy (meal, persona, relationship), you might want to take stock and reassess your priorities.

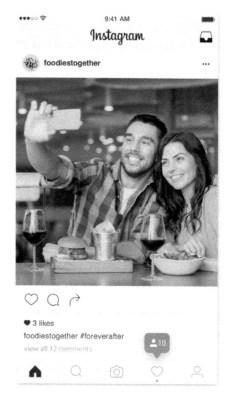

Immersion, the Counterweight to Excess

The best relationships develop when we give our undivided attention to our friends, family, and partners. Likewise, if we immerse ourselves in the process of eating we will get the most out of our relationship with food.

Have you ever arrived at a concert late? Or gone with a friend who was talking to you the whole time? Perhaps you were taking selfies and texting during the show? Maybe you had to leave early. When someone asks you, "How was that show? What songs did they play? What was the crowd like?" you struggle to give a detailed reply because you weren't entirely present.

Likely there was a period in your life when you had more free time and fewer obligations than you do now. In those carefree days you could go to a big event—a concert or football game—and relish every moment. Not only were you focused on the main attraction, but you found meaning in the details: the colors of the sky, the emotions of the crowd, a smile from a stranger, or the crackle of far-off thunder. Your commitment to the experience allowed you to savor every aspect.

When you watch a drum solo, seeing the drummer pound the shaking drum kit deepens your auditory experience. If you are in church listening to a sermon, the facial expressions and the body language of the preacher add potency and significance to the words. Meals are like any other multisensory event. What you get out of the occasion depends on the level of focus and attention you bring to it.

Consider all your senses while you eat. Are you devoting your eyes, ears, tongue, and nose to the experience, or is your attention elsewhere? When you immerse yourself, your eyes 'take photos' of the meal, your nose captures the aromas, and your taste buds record the incoming textures, tastes, and subtleties.

Ask not what your food can do for you…

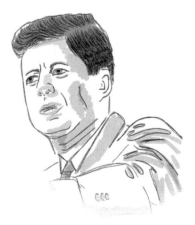

Allowing your senses to fully engage makes it easier for your brain to archive the memory. A detailed mental archive of meals improves your relationship with food and reduces cravings, binges, and poor meal choices.

When we are cutting calories we have to maximize every opportunity to enjoy our food and get the most MPC from every morsel. The guidelines that follow—on where, when, and how to eat—can help us reach those goals.

Where

You don't watch a movie in the bathroom and you don't take a nap on a treadmill. Likewise, though it is culturally permissible to chow down wherever we like, we are more immersed in eating when following these simple rules:

Do eat seated.	**Don't** stand and eat.
Do eat at your kitchen or dining-room table.	**Don't** eat at your desk, in front of your TV or computer, or in your bedroom.
Do eat in traditional meal settings: restaurants, cafés, workplace break rooms, etc.	**Don't** eat in the car, at your bus stop, on the subway, or on the street.

When: Appetite, Metabolism, and the Caffeine Diet

One summer day I met a group of weight loss clients in a shopping center for an educational tour of a grocery store. We had a long, relaxed breakfast at a restaurant and then strolled over to the nearby Whole Foods. I spent the next hour highlighting different foods and discussing their applications to weight loss. Midway through the tour one of my clients announced she was hungry, and by the end of the tour the entire group of five claimed to be starving. A similar phenomenon occurs when I teach classes on restaurant nutrition. I pass out menus to the students, who, no matter when they last ate, announce their hunger within minutes of studying the menu.

In both of those examples the word appetite should replace hunger. **Appetite** is the emotional desire for food. It comes from external influences: smelling pastries, seeing a late-night commercial for a juicy burger, hearing a catchy jingle, or having an intense conversation about food. Appetite can be stimulated whether the stomach is full or not, while hunger is a biological state. **Hunger** is inversely proportional to the amount of food in our gastrointestinal tract. Do not confuse these signals. Eat on your own schedule, independent from appetite cues.

Confusing appetite with hunger is not the only way to derail a healthy eating schedule. Caffeine can also do the trick. At La Clínica de La Raza, a health clinic I worked at in Oakland, California, I became accustomed to addressing the problems of the clinic's large population of overworked and obese Latino immigrants. Their stories fit a pattern that was surprisingly similar to the pattern of patients I've had across the socioeconomic spectrum:

A house cleaner with young children, Maria worked full time. The start of her day was always hectic. She rarely woke up feeling energetic, yet she had to get her kids off to school and arrive at work on time, leaving her little chance to get breakfast. It had been her habit to grab a pastry and coffee, but in recent years she'd become concerned about her health and switched to having fruit and yogurt with a large coffee. She was paid based on the number of houses she could get to, so she would only take a short lunch. She'd usually have another large coffee and a smoothie, sometimes adding in a taco or two, and an energy bar later in the afternoon. Though her workdays flew by in a caffeinated buzz of productivity she would feel exhausted and very hungry when she finally made it home. Once in the front door she'd plop on the couch and watch a telenovela to relax, and then it was off to snack in the kitchen while she prepared dinner. She'd then eat a large meal with her family: meat, rice, tortillas, cheese, salsa, and juice. Because of this large, late-day meal (which she often supplemented with late-night snacks), her busy digestive system disturbed her sleep and she would wake up the next day tired and with no appetite, thereby beginning the cycle anew.

Maria was surprised to learn that caffeine, like most stimulants, is an appetite suppressant. Drinking coffee in the morning and at lunchtime made less her hungry in the morning and early afternoon, but resulted in her snacking and eating heavier meals in the evening, after its effects wore off. To help her change this pattern I suggested that she brew slightly weaker coffee every day, and take more time to eat relaxed and balanced breakfasts and lunches that included energy-yielding carbohydrates like potatoes, corn, squash, and whole grains.

With this plan in mind we also negotiated a coffee compromise. She could drink a full, strong cup if it preceded exercise — in her case, Zumba class or walking. Maria started to associate a happy caffeine buzz with exercise, which led to regular and enthusiastic workouts. The adjustments to her eating, workout, and caffeine schedule had results: her appetite improved in the mornings and decreased at night, her weight dropped, and her energy level stabilized.

When you suppress your appetite with caffeine it rebounds with a vengeance.

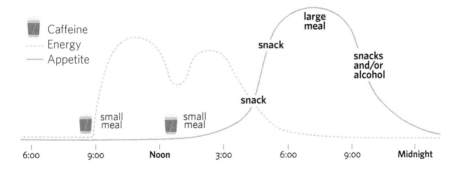

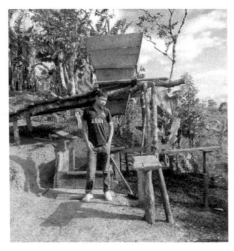

Coffee production wa established in most of Latin America by the mid-19th century.

Ivan, 14, works at the station where the pulpy shell of the coffee bean is removed. Nicaraguan coffee workers make $4 per day, which creates many challenges, including the ability to afford a nutritious diet. Most Nicas drink several cups of coffee a day, with one or two heaping tablespoons of sugar. Many children start drinking coffee almost from the moment they are weaned from breast milk.

(Barrio Nuevo, Madriz State)

In addition to disrupting our appetite's natural rhythm, our morning cup of joe affects our metabolism. At night our metabolism slows down and we burn calories at the slowest rate. Eating a breakfast of more than 300 calories — one that packs substantial volume and takes a solid half-hour to eat — breaks the fasting period and resets the metabolism to normal levels. Skipping breakfast, or eating a small or rushed breakfast, keeps our metabolism closer to the low nighttime levels and is likely to increase cravings later. Similarly, skipping or skimping on any meal increases the odds that our hunger will be out of control by the time we eat again.

No one should be famished by the time they have a meal. Breakfast should be eaten within an hour or two of rising. Lunch should be eaten no later than three to five hours after breakfast. Dinner should be eaten at least two hours before bedtime. Modest snacks between meals can help control your appetite. While the most important meal is breakfast, the late-afternoon snack can prove pivotal. It provides valuable fuel to complete the day's activities and prevents overeating at dinner. Note that the three-meals-plus-snacks pattern isn't the only approach; many people do well eating four or even six smaller meals a day.

Dr. Andrew Weil on stimulants (like caffeine): *"Do not take stimulants to help you perform ordinary functions. You should be able to get up in the morning, move your bowels, and make it through the afternoon without drugs."*[3] However, if you are going to use a drug, use it for the maximum benefit. With caffeine, exercise is an ideal outlet for the java high. Caffeine raises blood pressure, pulse rate, adrenaline, and dopamine, and most importantly gives the user an hour-or-two jolt of energy — all ideal effects for the demands of exercise.

How: Journaling

Although approaches to weight loss vary, maintaining a **diet journal** is one of the most universal features of effective diet programs for three reasons.

1   **Improved accounting:** You can only lose weight if you consume less than you burn, and this can only be verified by journaling your diet. Many calories go unaccounted because they are eaten mindlessly: the handful of M&Ms snagged from your friend's desk at the office, that energy bar you scarfed before a meeting, the dried pineapple chunks you snacked on while driving home. It's also easy to underestimate, misjudge portion size, and fail to account for invisibles (fats and sweeteners). By journaling you can see exactly where your calories come from. You can also fix weak moments—for example, you can bring carrot sticks to munch on in the car and replace those M&Ms with air-popped popcorn.

At the minimum your journal should include calories, portion sizes, and activity. Journal as often as you can. Many dieters do best when recording daily; aim for at least once a week. When you can't take time to record a meal, take photos and fill in the details later.

Journaling can be a challenge at first but gets easier as you become familiar with the calories in foods you commonly eat. Start by looking up calories and portion sizes on smartphone apps like My Fitness Pal or Calorie King; you can also carry a pocket-size calorie manual and a notebook. And don't stop at the numbers. Describe the environment of the meal: Was the TV on? Did you eat in the car? Were you relaxed and happy? Were you standing or seated? Did you eat cereal right from the box or did you use a bowl? Did your meal take 10 minutes or 40 to finish? You will find that all of this behavior is directly connected to your ability to feel full.

2   **Valuable biological feedback:** Use your journal to make notes on what I like to call "the four habits of the highly successful animal," namely, eating well, sleeping soundly, getting sufficient exercise, and moving your bowels at least daily. When these four habits are rountine the foundation for good health is strong. Note when you have a runny nose, fatigue, constipation or upset stomach, bad moods, colds, dry skin, rashes, headaches, and other nagging concerns. When these issues pop up take a look at your journal and see if there is a connection with your daily habits. Many patients discover **food allergies** this way. Pay attention to the feedback and adjust accordingly. Some common allergens to look for are dairy, gluten, sweeteners, and additives (such as monosodium glutamate, sulfates, and artifi-

cial colorings). The Center for Science in the Public Interest, a consumer advocacy organization, maintains a database on the most common food additives and their potential hazards. **Visit** cspinet.org/chemical-cuisine

Patients often ask me what they can do to improve **digestion.** They want to know if medications, supplements, or tests are needed to improve or detect deficiencies in digestive function. If you journal your digestive function you will likely notice that it correlates with both what you eat and how you eat. The latter starts with chewing. It is rarely acknowledged that the mouth is a crucial part of our digestive system. There are almost a dozen glands and ducts in the mouth that secrete enzymes and other digestive chemicals. When we eat too fast these digestive aids don't have time to do their job and our digestion suffers. When we pay attention to our meals, we chew more thoroughly and break food into smaller pieces. The smaller those pieces are, the easier it is for the stomach's acid to break down protein and for the enzymes of the small intestine to digest and assimilate the fats and carbohydrates.

3   **Promoting mindfulness:** Patients report that journaling gives them a sense of control. It helps them rewrite their story around food, health, and weight. Writing is a kinesthetic form of learning that can help us understand the process of dieting. The goal of immersion is to raise consciousness about an activity in which we often engage in a habitual, almost unconscious, state. Several of my Catholic patients tell me that monitoring reminds them of confession. Simply knowing they have to write everything down improves dietary habits, just as knowing they have to visit a priest on Sundays affects their choices during the week.

A diet journal is an ideal place to record weight. To ensure accuracy:

1   Check your weight at least once a week. Always weigh yourself first thing in the morning — weight fluctuates throughout the day.

2   Use the same scale every time. Scales vary, so periodically check your scale against one you know is accurate (e.g., at the doctor's office or at your gym).

3   Keep in mind the weight of your clothing. Belts, shoes, wallets, watches, and jewelry can affect measurement. Weigh yourself in your underwear or pajamas.

4   Be aware that a menstrual cycle will affect weight. Water weight can add several pounds.

How: Four Traits to Develop

Attention: You are an old-fashioned journalist, a food critic, with a wide-brim hat, a tweed suit, and a sharpened pencil. Every detail must be accounted for. Listen to the food. Does it make a pleasant crunching sound as you bite into it? Gaze at the colors of the food and inhale the varying smells. What textures are represented: smooth, brittle, thick, rough, sharp? How would you describe this to a painter so that he could re-create the scene before you?

Devotion: Eating is serious business, just as serious as sleep. Would you wake up at 3:00 A.M. to type out some work emails? No—and it's also not good to interrupt your meals. Think of the way an animal eats. If a dog is disturbed while eating, it growls or barks. Can you imagine a dog taking breaks from eating to howl at the moon or chase a rabbit? Animals give food their full attention, as should we.

Gratitude: You are on a desert island where your food choices are minimal. A crate washes ashore with a full meal on it. What luck! It might not be your dream meal but, like all food, it is a miracle. Savor this meal because who knows if another crate will wash ashore again.

Curiosity: Blindfold yourself during a meal (don't do this alone; have at least one other person at the meal who is not blindfolded). Do you notice anything different about the way you experience the meal? When you have one less stream of sensory information, your other senses become more acute and you can discern more subtle flavors. Fine restaurants play a similar trick with dim lighting and acoustics that soften sound.

....

Fewer distractions, more satisfaction

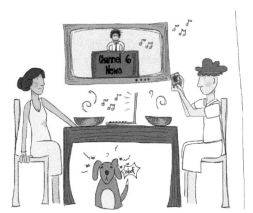 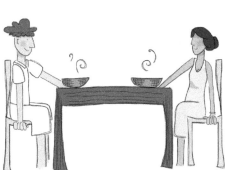

A Twelve-Step Program for Immersion

What follows is from a group activity I frequently lead in nutrition classes and weight loss workshops. I bring a basket of fruit and have students select one type. In a calm voice I read out loud the following instructions, pausing appropriately between steps. Try this at home with friends or family.

1   Take a full minute to **admire** the color, shape, and texture of the fruit. Are the surface texture and the color consistent? Is it smooth, or bruised?

2   Close your eyes and **imagine** where the fruit came from. Did it grow on a vine, a bush, or a tree? What did it look like when it was growing? Can you picture it? In what regions of the world can this fruit grow?

3   Can you **picture the climate** that nourished this fruit? The rainy spring that birthed it, the warm summer days during which it rapidly grew, and the cool, crisp fall day it was picked?

4   Bring the fruit beneath your nose and slowly **inhale and exhale** three times. Squeeze or pinch the fruit and breathe in the fragrance once more. Did the pressure affect the aroma?

5   Before putting the fruit in your mouth, imagine you're a journalist, eating the last piece of fruit on earth. **Savor** every morsel. Imagine writing an account of the experience so vivid that future generations could understand what it was like.

6   **Take one bite**, but do not begin chewing. Clear your mind; empty out all of the ideas running through you and bring your focus to the fruit that now sits in your mouth. Meditate on anything that comes to mind about its taste, texture, temperature, and note other sensations. Is the fruit consistent, or does it have variations in flavor and texture?

7   **Slowly begin chewing**, but do not swallow. If your thoughts wander off, bring them back to the process of chewing. **Notice** the movements of your jaw, the muscles in your head, and the way your teeth, tongue, and the fruit interact. Do you favor one side of your mouth?

8   How does chewing affect the flavor? Does it also affect the aroma? Can you still smell the fruit?

9   **How is this different** from drinking the juice of this fruit or eating a dried version of the fruit?

10 Before you swallow, make an intention to **follow the transition** from chewing to swallowing.

11 As you swallow, follow the fruit moving toward the back of your mouth and down your throat. Follow it until all sensation of the fruit disappears.

12 **Breathe** in deeply, exhale, and open your eyes.

How was this experience different from a typical bite of food? What did you notice while chewing? How much digestion occurred in your mouth? Was the food no longer tasty? Did it dissolve? Were you bored? Of course it is not recommended that you consume every bite of food this thoroughly. However, the exercise serves as a useful reminder about the power of immersion.

NOTES

1　Frederick Kaufman, "Debbie Does Salad," *Harper's*, October 2005, 58

2　Dr. Norman Doidge. *The Brain That Changes Itself* (New York: Viking Penguin, 2007), 102-112.

3　Winifred Rosen and Andrew T. Weil, *From Chocolate to Morphine: Everything You Need to Know About Mind-Altering Drugs* (Wilmington, MA: Mariner Books, 2004), 65

CHAPTER 10

Are We What We Eat?

Dietary Identity From the Roots to the Shoots

SEVERAL THOUSAND YEARS AGO A FEW OF OUR HUNTER-GATHERER ANCESTORS shifted from a nomadic way of life to the stability of farming. While the first farmers lived in small groups and retained the classless social system of hunter-gatherers, the seed had been planted for a future with far denser human populations and far more complex social systems. In *An Edible History of Humanity*, Tom Standage describes the ensuing developments: "An important step along the road from egalitarian village to a stratified city seems to be the emergence of 'big men' who win the control of the flow of surplus food and other goods and so amass a group of dependents or followers."[1]

The big men, formerly tribal chiefs and village elders, became leaders of thousands. Gradually, loose affiliations grew into formal hierarchies and, eventually, organized states. States supported agrarians by promoting the division of labor (adding layers to the hierarchy), recognizing property rights, and sponsoring public works: structures to store the harvest and irrigation projects to increase productivity. Farmers embraced empirical strategies: experimentation with plant and animal breeding; varying calculations for seeds, soil types, and acreage; rotation of crops; and schedules for planting, watering, and harvesting that co-evolved with the development of calendars and astronomy. While most hunter-gatherers retained the oral tradition of storytelling and spoke only in the present tense, the demands of agrarian life pushed language structures to develop past and future tenses, the use of symbols, numbers, and alphabets, mathematics, and the first written languages.

When the increasingly complex farming societies looked at their neighbors and saw people living in small bands, foraging in an untilled landscape, they no longer identified with their nonagrarian neighbors, regarding them as akin to wild animals. To the hunter-gatherers, geometrically arranged rows of crops, gentle domesticated animals, and densely populated, permanent human settlements were also profoundly foreign, as New York City might appear to an early agrarian. As agrarian societies flourished they appropriated land from traditional peoples—absorbing, enslaving, or killing them. Over thousands of years this trend resulted in our modern world, totally dominated by agrarians.

This pivotal fork in humanity's path relates to weight management in two ways covered in this chapter. It created the first distinct **diet-based identities**, and it made us **reconsider the meaning of status**.

Dietary Identity on a National Scale

As agrarian societies spread around the globe, their people characterized and distinguished themselves (and others, sometimes disparagingly) by the foods they most commonly produced and ate. The Maya called themselves "walking corn," the Japanese referred to Koreans as "garlic eaters," and the English called the sauerkraut-loving Germans "krauts."

The United States should call itself "the best potluck party on earth." Our dietary identity is shaped by two related factors: immigration and abundance. Immigrants came to America with their own dietary traditions: beloved special-occasion foods traditionally eaten only to celebrate holidays and major life events and simpler foods for everyday sustenance. As these new Americans became wealthier, they began to indulge in special-occasion foods much more frequently, and their staple foods became Americanized.

For instance, in Italy, a traditional pizza was a thin, salad-plate-size flatbread with modest layers of tomato and cheese and thinly sliced vegetables. In America, the size and thickness of pizza have grown exponentially; meat, cheese, and other calorie-rich toppings are piled high. Likewise, traditional Mexican tacos are small, with a few tablespoons of beans, meat, onions, and salsa, and rarely much dairy. In America, tacos are overstuffed with meat and dairy.

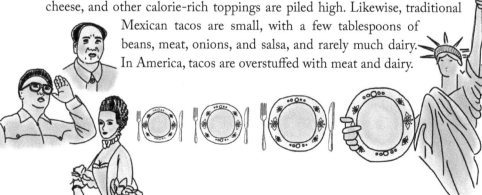

Asian dishes have also been remade to double or triple the portions of meat while reducing the vegetable component.

The use of food to celebrate abundance has a particularly poignant relevance in the United States. Many immigrants fled countries that used access to food as a political weapon. In Maoist China, Nazi Germany, Stalinist Russia—or any of dozens of repressive 19th- and 20th-century nations—dissenters were physically weakened, intimidated, and defeated by restriction of their access to food or even by intentional starvation. Unfortunately, these patterns of repression still exist. Many of my immigrant patients tell me they came to America so that they would never go hungry again.

Our collective memory of an impoverished past (our immigration stories, two world wars, the Great Depression) strengthens the lingering connection between modest diets and repression. As U.S. populations shifted from scarcity to abundance, excess calories became as much a part of our identity as the Stars and Stripes. "No one should go hungry in America" is a deeply seated value that bridges all political divides. It

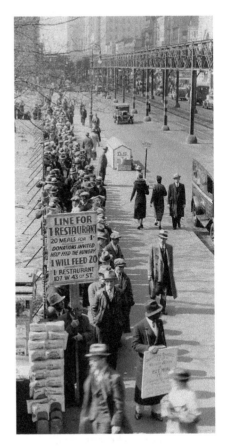

New York City's Midtown Manhattan, a center of unparalleled growth and wealth in the 1920s, hosts bread lines during the years of the Great Depression. Here, a sign advertises meals for 1¢ and requests donations.

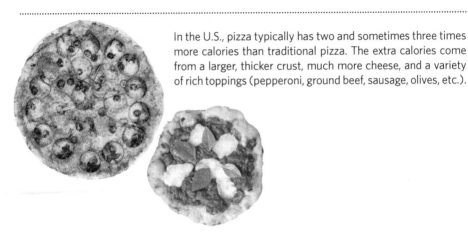

In the U.S., pizza typically has two and sometimes three times more calories than traditional pizza. The extra calories come from a larger, thicker crust, much more cheese, and a variety of rich toppings (pepperoni, ground beef, sausage, olives, etc.).

shares the same sacred footing as freedom of speech and religion. The government fights hunger through programs such as Women, Infants, and Children (WIC), the National School Lunch Program, and the Supplemental Nutrition Assistance Program (SNAP). Thousands of civic, religious, and secular charities also provide food assistance to the needy.

What's Cooking On the Stereo?

In post-Civil War America, traditional African music blended with the popular music of the era to give birth to jazz. In jazz, only the skeletal structure of the music is scripted. Via creative interpretations of rhythm and harmony, musicians rewrite the song with every performance. The apex of the improvisation is the solo, which frequently surpasses the melody in both length and importance. The result is that the same song sounds different with every rendition. This freedom of expression contrasted with Europe's classical tradition. In classical music, there was a strict hierarchy of composers, directors, and players, whose obligation was to perform music as written.

In the Old World, a repetitious dietary script based on nationality functioned like a classical music score. It varied little from year to year and encouraged faithful allegiance, not improvisation. American cooks, unbound by Old World strictures, were at liberty to mix influences from around the globe. In both food and music, American culture was defined by freedom, and the resulting indulgent expressions bathed the senses. Early critics of jazz warned that the wild music would overstimulate the listeners and lead to lewd and uncontrollable behavior. Although the warnings against "auditory excess" proved baseless, we can recognize the effects of gustatory excess.

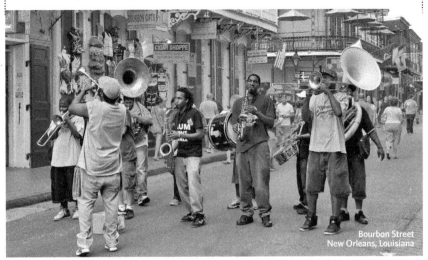

Bourbon Street
New Orleans, Louisiana

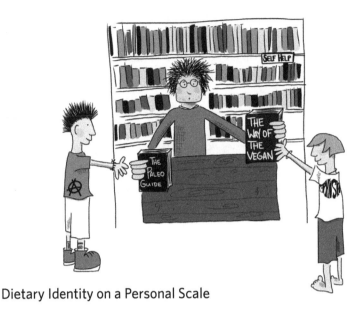

Dietary Identity on a Personal Scale

Patients often tell me it's challenging to change habits because they were raised in cultures that take pride in calorie-rich foods like heaping piles of pasta, rice, tortillas, cheese, meat, fried foods, and sweets. No culture celebrates steamed broccoli. It has been the nature of culture to promote foods that keep populations thriving while they work in physically demanding occupations. This cultural legacy still exists in the U.S., although fewer and fewer American occupations demand a high level of physical movement.

It is also the nature of culture to use food as a way to identify social classes. Are you a fast-food person? Or are you a slight step up, perhaps an Olive Garden or Ruby Tuesday aficionado? Are you a steak-and-potatoes macho man or a vegan-raw supermodel? Or have you ascended to such a pinnacle that your meals are trophies in the food rat race—each boosting you higher into the social stratosphere? Do they allow you to showcase your knowledge of culinary history, trends, and etiquette? Have you filled your home with sophisticated kitchen appliances, learned obscure techniques, and sought after rare, expensive ingredients?

Perhaps philosophy trumps status and you believe in the Paleo diet or its ethical opposite, the animal-loving vegetarian diet. Or you're a foodie who devours Michael Pollan books, Mark Bittman articles, and the traditional, wholesome meals they promote. Maybe you identify with your cultural or regional heritage via diet: a loyal Southerner who takes pride in home-cooked fried chicken, grits, and sweet tea; or an Italian who understands wines, cheese, and pasta.

Although some Americans still identify with a diet reflective of their heritage, we are increasingly untethered to tradition and bounce between food identities. Like a teenager who is a punk rocker one year and a hippie the next, we explore dietary options as a way of expressing ourselves.

You Can Take the Diet Out of the Country...

In nutrition the French paradox is famous: a relatively slim, healthy population can eat an enviable diet of cheese, bread, pastries, and wine. "Why can't that work for me?" you think.

The day-to-day lives of the French are markedly different from those of Americans. Visit Paris and you will find stunningly expensive gasoline, near constant bumper-to-bumper traffic, and scarce parking. While unaccommodating to cars, Paris, like most French cities, is pedestrian friendly with small, intimate streets and plenty of public squares, parks, bike paths, and public transportation. Whether home is a bustling metropolis or a quiet village, most French people live in close proximity to shops, work, and extended family, perhaps making child care and other obligations of life less stressful. Less dependent on cars than Americans, they spend a good deal more time walking and biking. They cook at home more frequently, eat comparatively slowly, have a deeply ingrained commitment to moderation in portion size,[2] and use far fewer pharmaceuticals per person than North Americans do. It is the sum of these differences that allows them to eat a fairly rich diet and maintain lower weights than Americans.

To follow, eating like a hunter-gatherer works fantastically well if your lifestyle follows suit: a great deal of physical activity and periodic fasts (or, as they used to call involuntary fasting in the good old days: starvation). Pollan and Bittman share the Paleos' rose-colored view of the past. These literary bards of the foodie movement inspired millions to consider the flaws of, and find alternatives to, our industrial food system. However, in their enthusiasm to turn back the clock to organic, pre-World War II foodways they often promote the traditional meals of that era—which, while minimally processed, are too calorie dense to facilitate weight loss. You can't butter your veggies like a 19th-century farmer if you aren't up at dawn milking cows or piling up hay bales. *The effects of diet cannot be isolated from their context: lifestyle, community, era, and culture.*

Status and Aspirational Societies

Part One: Shifting Identifiers in the United States (Eat Like a Boss)

In much of the world strict class systems define socioeconomic status. The USA is a rare country where, though inexcusable obstacles remain, some degree of class fluidity exists. Identity is flexible; one can aspire to any station in life. Though the uphill journey to the next social class is most often achieved via hard work, connections, luck, and education, the transition is marketed as attainable via consumption. Wear the clothes of the boss, become the boss! Eat pricey, sophisticated food; become a rich, sophisticated person! *In truth, despite our social mobility, consuming a sophisticated diet makes you no more sophisticated than consuming a French diet makes you French.* Sophistication comes from decades of acquiring skills, developing talents, and accruing accomplishments, not from patterns of consumption.

Young people seem to be most vulnerable to the myth of "eating your way to sophistication." According to an analysis of the Bureau of Labor Statistics' 2012 consumer expenditure survey, the amount of annual income that Americans younger than 25 spent dining out increased nearly 26 percent between 2000 and 2011. For ages 25 to 34, the increase was nearly 20 percent. This is particularly remarkable when one considers the economic stagnation of that decade. In a 2013 Washington Post article,[3] author Chris Richards noted a shift from people using music to identify and entertain themselves to using food for the same purpose: "today's gastronomical adventures provide the thrills that rock-and-roll used to." The article also quotes Kyle Rees, then communications manager at the Restaurant Association of Metropolitan Washington: "Cuisine exists in a cultural realm where people can engage in status displays and status items are things that aren't easily obtained. So if everyone can get music, it loses that value. [...] And the millennial generation, they're willing to drop the better part of their already low salaries on new food experiences."

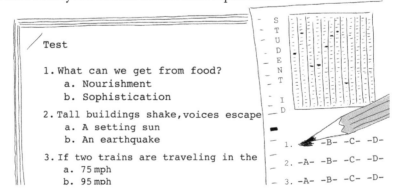

```
Test

1. What can we get from food?
   a. Nourishment
   b. Sophistication

2. Tall buildings shake, voices escape
   a. A setting sun
   b. An earthquake

3. If two trains are traveling in the
   a. 75 mph
   b. 95 mph
```

Part Two: Nicaragua — Out with the Old, in with the New

Western-style aspiration, in the form of the first U.S.-style retail stores, arrived in Nicaragua's cities in the 1940s and '50s. Refrigerators, telephones, radios, televisions and other goods were highly sought after. Nicaragua, like much of the developing world, began to look to the U.S. as the mecca of quality and innovation, and imported goods took on far higher status than local ones. Generally, this was logical: a light bulb casts more light than a candle, an electric drill is faster than a screwdriver, a truck hauls more than a donkey.

A similar thing happened with food. Foreign brands grew to represent status, sophistication, and wealth. In Nicaragua, a McDonald's or Wendy's is considered a place to celebrate big occasions — you might even ask your girlfriend to marry you at Pizza Hut. The power of the Western brand makes it hard for those of us who work in public health to persuade Latin Americans that indigenous staples such as beans, corn, and vegetables are better choices than burgers and pizza, and that water is healthier than sweet drinks. The challenge is explaining not only that what seems like a reliable axiom — the more modern the option, the greater the benefit — doesn't apply to food and diet, but that the relationship is usually inversely proportional.

In Nicaragua processed food and chronic disease have grown up together. Both rare only a generation ago, they are now pervasive. Two comments from my diabetic patients stay with me: "Imported breakfast cereals are better than local foods. They have more nutrients — it says so on the box!" and "The U.S. is the richest, most powerful country, so their food must also be the best."

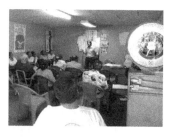

Above
The author working with diabetic patients at Hospital Roberto Huembes, Managua

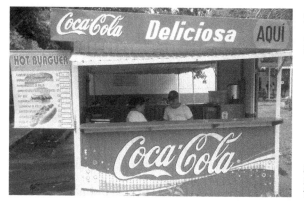

Left
A typical Nicaraguan fast-food stand

The Cyclical Definition of Status

If eating expensive or sophisticated food helps one acquire at least the facade of success and culture, there is a quality of an attractive person that *can't* be easily purchased: fitness. Most character flaws (dishonesty, vanity, gossiping) go unnoticed by passersby. No one is flawless, but the overweight have the misfortune of a visible shortcoming. Obesity is the new scarlet letter. The bias is well documented: the obese earn less money, have smaller social networks, marry less, have fewer children, and are more likely to suffer from chronic disease, depression, and other mental hea;lth issues. This bias, while cruel, has evolutionary roots. This brings us to the second consequence of the transition to agriculture: the ever-evolving definition of success.

Hot Hunters and Pudgy Bourgeois

The medium (in this case, the body) has always been the message. We evolved to find fitness attractive. In the hunter-gatherer era fitness increased the probability of survival and reproduction, making us better able to resist disease, escape predators, and obtain food. For the comparatively egalitarian hunter-gatherer, fitness was status, the primary metric for success. A shift occurred when agricultural and industrial societies developed. Possession of the means of production — land or factories — became the new yardstick for success. Hard physical work and meager resources kept farm and factory laborers slim, often to the point of malnourishment. A slim body became associated with poverty and disenfranchisement. Excess weight became the status symbol, indicating you'd risen above the toiling classes.

Only the Healthy and Wealthy Thrive

As the complex technological era supplants the agricultural and industrial past, changes are again afoot. Technology has created cheap calories and sedentary lifestyles, resulting in an epidemic of chronic disease and a scarcity of fitness. The fit minority, in a touch of circular history, again enjoy higher status, this time admired for their ability to outrun disease instead of predators. Adding to its allure, fitness is also highly correlated with education and income. Do money and smarts melt inches?

"You're looking fat!"
This used to be a compliment in much of the developing world. Now, as the majority has gone from thin to thick, excess weight has lost its appeal. After all, inherent in the definition of status is that it is not easy to obtain.

Achieving physical health can involve negotiating a labyrinth of illusions, tricks, dead ends, and outright scams. The privileged have the education to navigate at least some of this maze* and, when their efforts fall short, the money to invest in the healthcare professionals (doctors, dietitians, therapists, personal trainers) who can get them back on track.

* Indeed, it is a certain niche of highly educated people who design these traps, some of which are described in the next section.

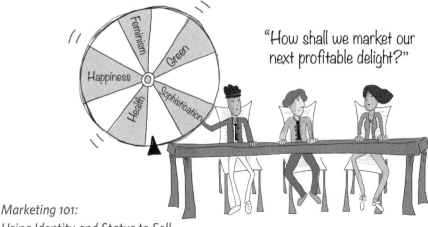

Marketing 101:
Using Identity and Status to Sell

What does that old adage "you are what you eat" mean? It means that we are the sum of the nutrients we eat. It does *not* mean we are the sum of the accolades awarded to the prestigious restaurants we frequent or the gourmet food we consume. Marketers exploit this misunderstanding with **five common tricks** that all have the same goal: to grant us permission; to provide us with a pretext for making a purchase.

1. **The Sophistication Ruse.** Since education is associated with success, it is valuable to cultivate a knowledgeable appearance. Food that is expensive, rare, imported, trendy, or superfluous (or harvested, processed, or prepared in a complex manner) increases the perceived value. Examples are craft beer, truffles, ostrich burgers, cauliflower-crust pizza, and kelp pasta.

2. **The Health Cloak.** Be wary of health claims: "high in antioxidants," "gluten free," "contains probiotics," "high fiber," "low cholesterol," "heart healthy," "low carb," high in this or that nutrient, etc. While these claims might all be true, they are rarely related to weight loss. Even most processed, calorie-dense foods are able to boast of one or two healthy-sounding qualities. *Don't confuse good for you with good for weight loss.* For weight loss, a surplus of nutrients is far less important than a deficit of calories.

3. **The Greenwash.** There is a plethora of fattening food that employs activism as a disguise. Our dollar is our vote and the world changes a little with every choice we make. However, buying organic chocolate-covered coffee beans harvested by a women's cooperative in Guatemala is not nearly as eco-friendly, or as healthy, as buying locally grown, unprocessed fruits, vegetables, fish, meat, dairy, legumes, and grains.

4. **The Happy Ploy.** Next time you see an ad, pay attention to the emotions of the people pictured. You'll see a common trend: food depicted as creating a positive emotional change. Think about how many ads feature frustrated, sad, or tired people whose moods improve magically after they eat or drink a product. In addition to the drug-like powers advertising promotes, there is another motive: those smiling happy people, jingles, contests, prizes, stories, and movie tie-ins are all intended to make us emotionally connected to specific brands.

5. **The Sister Act.** When processed foods were first introduced, the convenience of being able to open a can or box and have dinner ready in minutes was marketed as liberation for the modern woman. In recent decades all manner of rich food has been sold to women as a reward (edible trophies!) and as a way to rebel against the pressure to be slim. If dieting is equated with subjecting oneself to the patriarchy's narrow beauty standards, then eating rich food, no matter the consequences, can easily be marketed as an act of empowerment. Another segment of marketing is devoted to convincing men that certain calorically rich delights are inherently manly.

If you think these are the latest tricks from Madison Avenue, you are probably not familiar with the history of lobster. In the 17th and 18th centuries lobster was considered inedible, unsanitary, and so downright repugnant that some states, citing cruel and unusual punishment, limited the number of times per week lobster could be fed to inmates. A few clever New Englanders realized that many Midwesterners, never having seen a lobster, had no such prejudices. Two developments greased the wheels: the expanding railroad networks of the 19th century dropped transportation costs, and the fairly new concept of newspaper advertising (and increasing literacy rates) allowed for the reshaping of the previously maligned crustacean's identity as an exotic, expensive specialty.

Not only can marketing shape our perception of status, but it can also mold our overall view of food's role. Food marketing has led us to pile on multiple roles for food: identity, emotional support, status, medication, friend, enemy, reward and punishment. (Could *you* raise three kids, work full time, take care of your mother-in-law, learn Chinese, and volunteer at a senior citizen's home?) When we push external values on food we also attach external reasons to eat. How we perceive food is flexible, so why not actively shape our perception in ways that help us reach our weight goals? *It is time for food to return to its original purpose: nourishment to fuel life.*

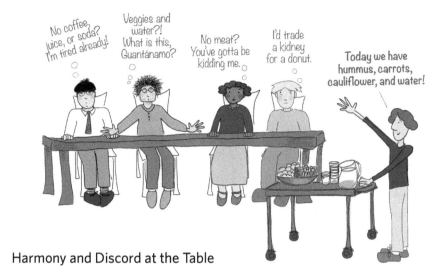

Harmony and Discord at the Table

"After a good dinner one can forgive anybody, even one's own relations."

OSCAR WILDE

Let's consider a working-lunch office meeting. What foods do you expect to be served? Typical fare is cheese and crackers; soda, juice, and coffee; sandwiches or pizza; and cookies or pastries for dessert. People often come to meetings feeling anxious, tired, stressed, or combative. They are both soothed and stimulated by the snacks. These pleasures are the lubricants of our hectic society, delivering the grease that minimizes social friction and keeps the wheels turning. We bond over calorie-dense foods in much the same way that we bond over drugs and alcohol. We might acknowledge that a certain food or drug is bad for our health but indulge nevertheless. In most social situations indulging is "cool"—it indicates to others that we're relaxed people who seek easy pleasures and won't judge others for doing the same.

Possibly the most common type of pressure we get is a simple nudge: "You've got to enjoy life!" That rationalization slips out just before the burger or beer slips in. Sharing the same food unites people. When we gather to share meals a discerning eater is often perceived as choosing not to identify with the group, and might get characterized as a health nut, picky, difficult, self-centered, or narcissistic. It is a primal impulse to cast out the nonconformist. When you're trying to lose weight, this phenomenon can sabotage success.

Another way we give ourselves a cover to indulge is to mimic, perhaps unconsciously, the marketers: "I made these cheeseburgers using only the best—grass-fed beef and artisanal cheddar," or "This smoothie has antioxidant-rich açaí berries from Brazil."

Don't take it personally. *Be patient*—struggles with weight are common, and as you progress you will find more supporters than detractors. In the meantime it is good to have a tactful response or two at the ready. This can be nothing more than the humble truth: "I *am* working on enjoying life by getting in shape. These treats are stumbling blocks for me." One client of mine uses comedy as a response. Grabbing her love handles, she counters with "I *have* enjoyed everything—and here's the proof!"

It is naive to hope that we can entirely separate diet from identity. However, it is possible to develop an identity independent from marketers, in which we define ourselves by our commitment to well-being. Consider the time and money spent on hairstyles and fashion choices, both of which are considered central to expressing individuality. No one berates you for making a spirited effort to look your best, so don't think twice about reinventing your diet and lifestyle to improve your health and yes, perhaps, tweak your identity.

Teaching Balance. Bell Gadea, one of my nutrition students from the National Autonomous University of Nicaragua, is a member of the student group Vida en Equilibrio (Life in Balance). She and her group conduct workshops in poor communities, teaching about healthy, affordable diets based on local foods. They also demonstrate and teach activities like yoga, aerial silks, and slacklining. (*Somoto*)

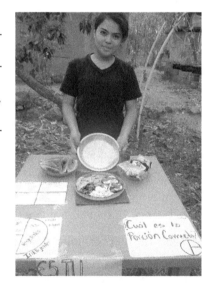

NOTES

1 Thomas Standage. *An Edible History of Humanity* (New York: Walker & Company, 2008), 53.

2 In 1904 France passed a public health law creating clinics to teach nutrition—with an emphasis on portion control—to mothers. Over time, portion control became a central component of French public health policy and was widely applied in schools, hospitals, and other institutional settings. Even outside official settings portion control was widely adopted and became a defining pillar of French cuisine at home, at restaurants, and at work. Barry M. Popkin, *The World Is Fat* (New York: Avery Publishing, 2009), 38-39.

3 Chris Richards, "Are Foodies Quietly Killing Rock and Roll?" *The Washington Post*, May 10, 2013.

CHAPTER 11

The Wallet and the Scale

SOME PEOPLE CONSUME MATERIAL GOODS WHEN STRESSED, some consume calories, and some do both.

A Siesta From the Rat Race

I met Cecilia and her husband, Sherman, while I was running a weight loss program at Rancho La Puerta, a green wellness resort. Cecilia and Sherman owned and ran a small tech company. In the late 1990s their company prospered, and they became accustomed to an upper-class lifestyle. The couple and their twin girls lived in a beautiful house in a fashionable suburb on the California coast. They drove late-model cars and had attractive furniture, elegant artwork, fashionable clothes, and an entertainment system that reached every nook of the house. In the 2000s, as the tech industry became more competitive, they had to work harder to land clients and their workload climbed to more than 50 hours per week.

Cecilia had struggled with her weight for about a decade. Having seen several dietitians, she had a strong understanding of nutrition. She had tried a succession of well-planned approaches to diet, but she had never been able to make them stick. Her case seemed—at first—to be an instance of someone who was making sensible choices but still couldn't get the scale to budge.

Another piece of the puzzle came when Sherman confided in me that he worried that they were living beyond their means. He described a typical shopping trip: "Cecilia bought several hundred dollars' worth of clothes for our three-year-old twins. What's the point? The girls don't care if they are wearing thrift shop clothes or Ralph Lauren. I know she wants to show how much she loves them, but sometimes I think she just loves to shop."

I was still pondering Sherman's words a few hours later when the couple offered to give me a ride into town. As Cecilia raised the back seat of their small sports car to make room for me, she made an unpleasant discovery. Clutching a crumpled leather jacket in her hand, she turned to her husband and angrily barked, "Look at it—just look at it! This was your Father's Day present! A $400 jacket—and what do you do with it? No wonder I never saw you wear it."

Cecilia came to the resort primarily focused on her weight, but I concluded that her obesity was only partly due to her eating habits. She worked all the time, didn't exercise much, was constantly stressed, and didn't sleep well. Dining out and shopping sprees were the only outlets she allowed herself.

My first strategy for Cecilia was to help her find ways to reduce her expenditures, which in turn would allow her to work fewer hours and create a healthier, more balanced lifestyle. While we worked together we covered stress management, reviewed healthy eating and sleep habits, and studied her spending habits to determine what was essential and what could be reduced or eliminated.

The case I made for significant lifestyle change was bolstered by Cecilia's experience at the resort. For the first time in years, she mindfully ate three balanced meals a day and, most importantly, slept soundly every night. She went on daily hikes and enjoyed a variety of fitness classes, all of which helped calm her restless body. She worked on calming her restless mind by reawakening her creative side in a series of art workshops. The lack of sedentary entertainment at the resort (no TV and only limited internet access) gave her time to practice her commitment to reducing her workload. She continued to telecommute three or four hours a day, but that was far less than her usual ten-hour workday.

Cecilia dropped more than 10 pounds during her stay. Back at home, she continued to reduce her financial stress and workload. She made time for physical activity and her energy picked up. She focused on rewards other than shopping, and her cravings declined accordingly. About six months after her stay she emailed to let me know she'd reached her goal weight.

The top two reasons for lack of sleep:

1. Our bodies, our actual muscles, are restless. They haven't moved much in the day and they can't relax at night.
2. Our minds are restless: too many thoughts, worries, and concerns prevent us from letting go.

Stress

"What you feel when life's demands exceed your ability to meet those demands."
DR. SHAWN TALBOTT

Stress's role in disease and weight gain has been comprehensively explored. Here is a brief summary of the scientific consensus.

Throughout human history almost all the stress we experienced was physical. When our lives were endangered we had two options: to run away or to stand and combat the threat. (You may be familiar with the scientific term "fight or flight" response.) Threats trigger the release of hormones, most significantly **cortisol**. Cortisol increases blood sugar, blood pressure, breathing rate, and heart rate; it also redirects our circulation from our internal organs to our muscles. These effects are ideal for physical activity. If you have ever had a close call, you are familiar with the electric spike of alertness and energy that proximity to danger unleashes.

In our evolutionary past, most stressors arose and faded quickly. Cortisol spiked, then rapidly dissipated after the burst of activity ended. The mechanism at fault in modern life is that psychological stress triggers the same response as physical stress. When psychological stress is brief and occasional, the body recovers quickly. Unfortunately, modern stresses like financial struggles or the long daily commute can peck away at us over months and even years. Chronic stress creates a long-term hormonal imbalance in which chronically elevated cortisol levels have many consequences. These can include:

1   Signaling the body to refuel after responding to a stressor, resulting in an amplified appetite. The more stress, the more persistent the appetite.

2   Increasing our resistance to the hormone insulin, which leads to fluctuations in blood sugar, increased cravings, and additional fat storage.

3   Increasing the efficiency at which we turn calories into fat, especially the visceral fat that pads our abdominal region.

4   Decreasing testosterone levels—testosterone helps both men and women build and maintain muscle mass.

It's not enough to simply eat well and exercise. The best weight loss plans must include a stress management component.

Something's Got to Give

Cecilia's pattern was similar to that of many of my clients, people who had prioritized work (whether to achieve a goal such as a promotion or to start or keep a business running) to the detriment of their health. In addition to their own economic priorities, many felt responsible for the financial well-being of their fellow employees and, in some cases, investors.

It's an absurdly common decision to choose our work over our health. While financial benefits are tangible — *x amount of extra work equals x number of dollars* — the gradual erosion of our constitution is intangible and difficult to quantify. Many of us don't see a downside until a serious illness or other crisis forces us to reassess our priorities and our lifestyle.

Correspondingly, living beyond our means can be a subtle form of self-destruction, whether it's by choice (keeping up with the Joneses) or by necessity (keeping the roof over your head).

A challenge inherent in changing our priorities is that putting good health before money is often regarded as selfish, even narcissistic. Money is the universal metric of our culture; everyone sympathizes with a decision to work more. Ironically, while investments in health come at a short-term cost the long-term result is often a more productive person — and worker.

Recall the descriptions of the Sober Plate in Chapter 3. The same balance, the same cause and effect, applies to work and health.

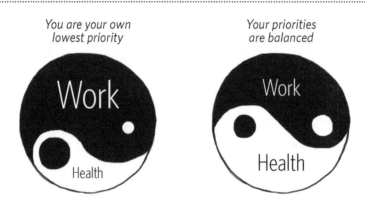

Work (all that is obligatory and requires effort): paid work, nonpaid work, commuting, errands, chores

Health (all that supports health): sleep, diet, physical activity, creative outlets, community, family, faith or spirituality

Might I Grind Your Pepper, Sir?

"Restaurants are to people in the '80s what theater was to people in the '60s"

"WHEN HARRY MET SALLY" (1989)

While I was working with Cecilia and Sherman on their fiscal and caloric budgets, they calculated that they routinely spent about $1,000 each month on meals eaten outside the home, most often at full-service restaurants. They both relished the feeling of being taken care of, as a reward for the long hours they worked, but they agreed that this was an expenditure that they were willing to reduce. I recommended that they reserve fine dining for a limited number of special occasions, do more cooking at home, and make a switch to "fast casual" restaurants.

We *don't* always have time (or want to make time) to prepare our own food, but fine dining, frozen meals, and fast food aren't the only options. Fast-casual restaurants offer meals that average under 10 dollars. While they offer some typical high-calorie menu options, they also offer low-calorie, healthy dishes. Chipotle, Sweetgreen, Baja Fresh, Cava Grill, Chopt, Protein Bar, Lyfe Kitchen, and Veggie Grill are examples of this trend.

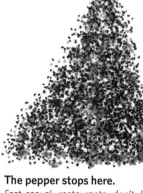

Cecilia and Sherman began to cook more regularly at home, replacing their go-to frozen fare with a handful of easy-to-prepare, healthy dishes. While they continued to eat about half their meals outside the home, the switch to fast casual allowed them to cut their monthly food expenditure by more than $600. A few months later Cecilia shared her insight about the change: "At first I missed the whole ritual: the tablecloth, the nice plates and silverware, having a waiter advise me on menu options, bring my food, and pour me water, but then I started to think maybe I'd been fetishizing eating by buying into the theatrics. I was paying extra to feel important and special. I don't want the artifice anymore; I can feel good in a more authentic way."

The pepper stops here.
Fast-casual restaurants don't have full table service, but they do offer higher-quality food than fast-food restaurants, and use fewer frozen or processed ingredients. You can usually expect nicer decor, fairer pricing, faster service, flexible offerings, and a full view of the food being prepared.

Finding the Balance

What Makes Change Possible?

Cecilia's quiet time at the resort allowed her to reflect: "I remember sitting in our cabin at Rancho La Puerta thinking, 'This body, this *life* is all I really own—but neither is in great shape.'"

When do people experience epiphanies, revelations, and transformations? Many journeys of self-discovery and change begin with a move or travel: a year abroad, walking the path of St. James, hiking the Appalachian Trail, a long road trip, or just a short journey such as Cecilia's.

Could you make a change similar to Cecilia and Sherman's? It can be hard to give up the cosmetic perks that come with a certain level of consumerism. Much as friends bond over food, social and class identification occurs through name brands and material goods. All you have to do is cruise through your neighborhood in your sports car, or have your nanny take your baby to the park in the high-end stroller, and you advertise what kind of money you're working with. Giving up that social shorthand can be temporarily painful; superficial friendships may dissolve. Knowing that, and knowing that authenticity and balance have their own rewards, can make the transition easier.

Cecilia's commitment to change made a huge difference in her life, her career, and her family. "After getting used to simpler food, it didn't seem so bad to not have the latest fashions. Now that I am feeling better about my body, I am less worried about what other people think of me. We even ended up selling the sports car. Thanks to less financial pressure I'm back down to a 40-hour workweek and I actually feel as productive as ever. With my new free time, I exercise, I play with my kids more, and I am having fun painting and gardening." Together with Cecilia and Sherman's other budget-cutting moves, their monthly expenditures dropped by well over $1,000 per month. Selling their sports car netted an additional windfall plus considerable monthly savings.

The curse of being lost in possessions is common in our shared mythology: Jacob Marley and Ebenezer Scrooge, Jay Gatsby, Charles Foster Kane and, perhaps the most dramatic example of all, Tolkien's Gollum. We recognize these archetypes as being dissolute, burdened, obsessed, and unable to enjoy life.

Possessions, a Two-Way Street

Why do you cherish your late grandmother's necklace, your autographed football jersey, your collection of vintage *Rolling Stone* magazines? We respect, even if we don't understand, the ability of objects to accrue not only monetary value but also emotional value. When we give our time to objects — searching for, purchasing, storing and caring for them, and looking to them for fulfillment — the objects begin to own us. The debt we then owe makes this more than a quaint philosophical theory: many of us are quite literally working to pay off our purchases.

While associating ourselves with possessions can become a way of disassociating from ourselves, a separation from possessions leaves us alone with ourselves. We feel like different people because our bodies are who we are without possessions.

I'm not suggesting we donate all of our worldly goods and don loincloths. Rather, we can seek a balance that removes the stress of living beyond our means.

We can see evidence that more people are seeking this balance in the rise of the sharing economy. Many are choosing to buy smaller homes and fewer (or no) cars. Nontraditional business models like Uber and AirBnB allow us to have the occasional luxury of a car or a vacation home, without the long-term financial burden.

Better Living Through Chemistry

"Everything's amazing right now, and nobody's happy."

LOUIS C.K.

The relationship among possessions, health, and weight goes beyond the philosophical. The explanation for shopping's and eating's therapeutic effects is well established: both trigger the brain to release chemical messengers called neurotransmitters, the most important of which is dopamine. Dopamine is a precursor of adrenaline and the closely related molecule noradrenaline, both of which trigger feelings of joy and excitement.

When we make a purchase we get a joyful jolt of dopamine from the brain. For a few days afterward, looking at our purchase will cause our brain to release more dopamine, but in steadily decreasing amounts. Think about the excitement over Christmas presents. How long does the buzz from that new phone, purse, or laptop last?

Dopamine is also released when we eat: the more calories, the more dopamine. As we increase consumption, however, our brain responds by reducing the number of dopamine receptors, making us less sensitive to dopamine's effect.

In other words, the buzz wears off quickly and we build up a tolerance. If we seek to achieve the same dopamine buzz as before, we need to increase the quantity we consume.

A vicious cycle develops: increased consumption results in less sensitivity (fewer receptors), and the appetite responds by rising to compensate. This cycle is remarkably similar to the cycle of diminishing returns that characterizes addiction to drugs like cocaine, heroin, and prescription painkillers. The reward we get from external sources (consumption) can become a substitute for natural sources of positive emotions.

Although we think of the feedback mechanism above as frustrating, perhaps even unfair, consider the results if overconsumption had no biological or social consequences. If drugs, rich food, and material possessions yielded ever-increasing returns of consequence-free bliss, our pleasure seeking would cause us to strip the earth bare and we would become a planet of battling Jabba the Hutts. In this light, the increasing consumption/diminishing returns physiological loop can be seen as one of the most important mechanisms in all of biology.

Outsmarting the Hedonic Treadmill

The nascent field of positive psychology, which studies what makes a happy life, describes the frustrating feedback loop as a **hedonic treadmill**: no matter what you buy or consume, the effect on your happiness is temporary and you eventually return to the same starting point. A lot of people I met at Rancho La Puerta were stuck on that treadmill: successful, with everything they needed, but still wanting more.

Positive psychologists conclude that once people's basic needs are met, excess does not bring any sustainable increase in well-being; they add that we are poor prognosticators of our own happiness. Accordingly, it is important that we develop the practices that allow us to lead a satisfying life. While the definition of "the good life" is subject to many interpretations psychologists have made a distinction in one critical aspect: emphasizing the difference between pleasure and gratification. **Pleasure** is primarily temporary and passive and subject to the treadmill's limitations. **Gratification** requires effort and sometimes discomfort, but its benefits are long term and are not subject to the feedback loop of diminishing returns.

Dr. Mihaly Csikszentmihalyi, a leader in the field, sums up the difference:

> "Pleasure is a powerful source of motivation, but it does not produce change; it is a conservative force that makes us want to satisfy existing needs, achieve comfort and relaxation…Enjoyment [gratification] on the other hand is not always pleasant, and it can be utterly stressful at times. A mountain climber may be close to freezing, utterly exhausted, in danger of falling into a bottomless crevasse, yet he wouldn't want to be anywhere else. Sipping a cocktail under a palm tree at the edge of the turquoise ocean is nice, but it just doesn't compare to the exhilaration he feels out on that freezing ridge."[1]

Indeed, the common belief that material wealth and indulgent food increase long-term happiness is mistaken. This thinking fails to take into account that the joy of consumption is fleeting. We adapt to our new conditions, and they become our new normal—not the state of permanent contentment we had hoped for. No one advises the avoidance of pleasure. Instead, pleasures should be occasional indulgences to be slowly savored, as opposed to a daily strategy to cope with reality.

A similar misconception acts as a barrier to engaging in physical activity, one of the primary examples of behaviors that bring long-term benefit. Many of us instinctively believe that most forms of physical activity are tedious or unpleasant. We put it off as long as we can or even avoid it altogether. In this case we don't account for some beneficial side effects of the body's natural release of neurotransmitters. Neurotransmitters triggered by an internal catalyst (moving our bodies), unlike those released by an external action (shopping or eating), are not subject to tolerance. In other words, if playing soccer or dancing for 45 minutes on Tuesday made you happy, you don't need 50 minutes to produce the same effect on Wednesday. Sports are one example of the natural high (you're probably familiar with the term "runner's high") inherent in physical activity; you can achieve similar benefits from creative pursuits (singing, playing music, making art) and different types of social contact (hugging, massage, intimacy). *Make gratification your goal.*

The research on the hedonic treadmill is an example of **a sea change in healthcare**: preventing disease by studying and supporting the factors that sustain mental and physical health, as opposed to treating patients only after disease has manifested. Dietitians are advising, "Skip the short-term pleasures of a rich diet and reap long-term health," and psychologists are counseling, "Limit the quick-fix pleasures; focus on habits that build gratification."

Monopoly and the Void

Our impulse to chase easy pleasures implies we have a void to fill. Perhaps emptiness is part of the human experience. Without that void we might still be content huddling by the Paleolithic campfire. For most of our species' history, filling the void was motivation to explore nonmaterial pursuits: sport, music, art, theater, literature, science, philosophy, and religion. The conclusion of psychologists is that we would benefit from a return to these activities: doing, rather than consuming.

Timothy Ferriss, in his bestseller *The 4-Hour Workweek,* takes on the subject from a different perspective. Ferris writes about the desires of the "new rich," who no longer prioritize material possessions and early retirement. Their goal is to "do all the things you want to do and be all things you want to be."[2] Ferriss elaborates on typical new-rich dreams of acquiring skills and experiences: traveling, learning to tango, living abroad, racing motorcycles, becoming a professional kickboxer. According to Ferriss, the central motivating question in life often is now, "What excites you?" It appears that at least some of the modern elite have adopted positive psychologists' ideas. In dozens of reality TV shows and tabloid magazines, we are encouraged to snicker at the bejeweled inanities of the rich who cling to idle consumerism: throwing tantrums because their new luxury car is the wrong shade of burnt sienna or dousing each other in champagne over insults about botched cosmetic surgery.

As we reevaluate traditional forms of wealth, the game of Monopoly as a metaphor for success must also evolve. Declaring a winner based solely on money no longer matches our widening understanding of a meaningful, contented life. Our new hero doesn't own all the hotels on the boardwalk; rather it is the sprightly grandmother who goes out for a morning jog, the gray-haired father who gives his teenage son a run for the money on the basketball court, the neighbor who paints away his blues instead of eating them. Even if you play by the old rules—you dress like a model and acquire high-status possessions—draw the line at what enters your body.

Every choice you make decides who the future you will be. This is sacred ground, and no commercial entity should tell you what to do. You work toward balance because you are grateful for your good health, vain enough to reap the rewards, and strong enough to make independent choices.

NOTES

1   Martin Seligman, *Authentic Happiness* (New York: Atria Books, 2003), 118.
2   Timothy Ferriss, *The 4-Hour Workweek* (New York: Harmony, 2009), 47.

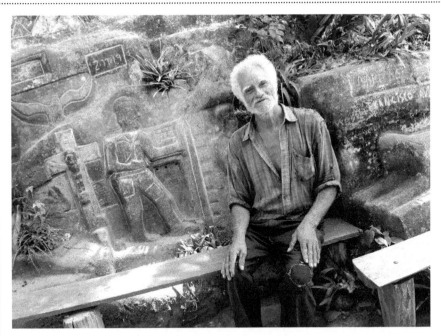

Converting Pain to Beauty

I met Alberto Gutiérrez Girón in 2006 while visiting the Tisey Estanzuela Natural Preserve in northern Nicaragua. Alberto told me that as a young man he developed a drinking problem. His priest advised him to find a hobby to help replace alcohol, so Alberto taught himself to sculpt. Alberto is now nearing 80 and has spent more than 40 years carving acres of mountainside in the preserve. He grows his own food and his home is a small cabin without electricity or running water. Despite the fact that he has never promoted or sold any of his art (it's all attached to the mountain), word of his work has spread all over the world. In an average month he gets 100 visitors, whom he happily guides on hikes to see his extensive works.

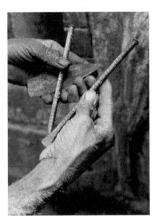

Alberto has reinvented the Monopoly game. Beautifying the world replaces buying hotels, inspiring others substitutes for collecting rent, and every time he passes "Go" he makes a few more friends.

Simple Tools Move Mountains: Alberto's only sculpting tools are sharpened pieces of rebar, a metal blade, and a stone hammer.

There is another photograph of Alberto's work on page 105.

CHAPTER 12

The Marketer, the Caveman, and the Priest

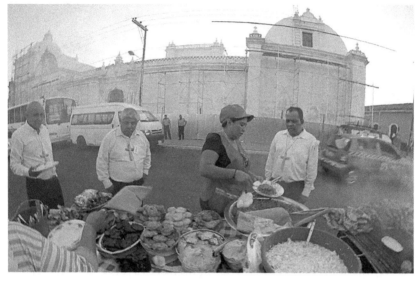

Priests fill up on fried food at the fritanga across the street from the church. (*Leon*)

THE CENTRAL OBSTACLE IN WEIGHT LOSS can be summed up as "Why can't I easily give up calorie-rich food?" In this battle, evolution has made us vulnerable on two fronts: our sensitivity to stimuli and our proclivity to excess.

Sensitivity to Stimuli

Humans evolved to absorb the meaning of everything in their environment. The ability to correctly interpret every sound, image, smell, texture, and taste aided survival. Are those clouds puffy and dark—*thunderstorm: take shelter!*—or light and scattered? Is that animal poised to strike or to flee? Is this the poisonous blood-red berry or the edible ruby-red one?

We have retained this evolutionary survival mechanism despite the fact that most of the stimuli to which we are now exposed (and to which we respond, much of the time unconsciously) aren't relevant to our survival, but instead are carefully designed to manipulate us.

Everything we absorb from our environment has an impact. In some cases we are conscious of the power of an external stimulus. We might visit a national park or museum, or attend a sporting or musical event, because we want to be influenced, even inspired, by the most affecting examples of what our senses can take in. Conversely, we might try to limit our exposure to (and prevent our children from experiencing) obscenity- or violence-filled music, images, and games. It's important to note, however, that persuasive exposure can take many forms. It can be powerful but intermittent—instances in which we've chosen the exposure—or constant but subtle. The subtle form consists of more passive messages (think about waste bins sporting "landfill" or "recycling" labels) that encourage us to think about the consequences of our actions.

The Marketer: Round-the-Clock Persuasion

"A man is what he thinks about all day long."
RALPH WALDO EMERSON

Have you ever wondered why your dentist's waiting room has a fish tank, soft music, and tranquil nature photographs? Why your favorite shops play music you like? Why fast-food restaurants have bright lighting and vibrant color schemes? These are all well-researched ways of using visual and aural stimuli to modify our behavior: to calm us down, to keep us happy and engaged while we shop so that we spend more time and money, or to cue us to eat up and vacate our seats for the next hungry customer.

Marketers specialize in detecting and manipulating the stimuli that influence our decision making. A fundamental law of marketing is that **exposure drives behavior**. The more exposure a brand has, the more sales increase. Aware that our sensitivity to stimuli is far greater than we realize, marketers now go beyond conventional advertisements to exploit more subtle ways to influence us.

In his book *Buyology*, Martin Lindstrom details the techniques of subliminal marketing. For example, Coca-Cola not only bought advertising time on the show "American Idol" but paid for a presence in the set design: the judges' chairs matched the distinctive curve of Coke's classic bottle, and the walls were Coke-brand red. Marlboro paid nightclubs to redesign their interiors, upholstery, tiles, and wallpaper to have patterns that mimicked the Marlboro logo.[1] In *Brandwashed*, Lindstrom describes working with a beverage manufacturer to design the shape of its can's pop-top to produce a unique sound. The manufacturer paid to broadcast this sound at public events. Amazingly, this trifling, intermittently played, one-second crackle and hiss of carbonation proved sufficient to spark an immediate spike in sales: within minutes, people lined up to buy the drink.[2] These examples are part of a larger trend in marketing that forgoes direct advertising. Companies need only remind us of an associated sound, shape, color, or pattern to prompt us to buy.

The same logic is at play when companies give away items branded with their corporate logo or theme. You can clothe yourself head-to-toe in logo-covered items, and drink, write, calculate, bag your groceries, freshen the air, dry off at the beach, light your way home, and hug a teddy bear—all while building your brand loyalty and passively advertising for Company X. Those T-shirts, thumb drives, flashlights, and pens are a calculated investment. Keeping the brand fresh in consumers' minds—and building positive associations—result in more sales, which easily exceed the cost of the freebies.

Self-Marketing

We tend to disregard claims that meditation reduces stress, that aromatherapy improves mood, or that posting positive images and messages can enhance optimism and productivity. In the commercial context we call influential messages marketing (think about Nike's "Just do it" campaign), but in the noncommercial context we underestimate our sensitivity. Don't be too cynical. We know how effective sales-oriented marketing is, and we can tap that power for our own benefit: **self-marketing** also works. You might already do some or all of these: listen to up-tempo music to quicken your step when you're working out; help yourself relax by playing soothing tunes and lighting a scented candle; inspire your diet and fitness efforts by taping a picture of a favorite athlete by your mirror. Self-marketing by omission works, too: when you want to lose weight, you don't go to all-you-can-eat buffets or walk down the candy aisle at the grocery store.

Actively select what you want to reinforce in your life. If you want to be healthier, support yourself with actions, images, and messages that encourage healthy choices in your home and work.

Consumer habits, like much of human behavior, are highly plastic. If we don't devise a conscious strategy to shape those habits ourselves, marketers—and our peers, whose habits are likely also shaped by marketers—will form them.

Power Politics and External Influences

Understanding that our behavior and choices are affected by outside influence is crucial. What we do with that knowledge is even more important.

We might be inclined to want to filter out every influence, but this is impossible: we don't make decisions in a vacuum. We know that there are overtly negative pressures to counter, but we can also be negatively affected by well-intentioned influences of our family and friends, our colleagues, years of habits, and peer pressure.

It's also not a great leap to regard some influencers with suspicion or even fear, especially large, well-organized entities (federal government agencies, the marketing efforts of big corporations, media outlets, world trade organizations). They can embody the worry that a relatively small segment of society wields undue influence over the day-to-day lives of ordinary people. In the U.S., the protest movements Occupy Wall Street and Tea Party Patriots made that worry the centerpiece of their opposition. Unlike traditional protests devoted to specific causes (antiwar, pro-environmental cleanup) or rights for specific groups (women, minorities, unions) these movements were about the loss of control. One group's concern was that the wealthiest one percent of society controlled the government; the other's concern was that federal government policy was interfering with personal liberty.

If we're going to regain power over our own lives, we can start by taking a more conscious approach to decision making. We can educate ourselves and think critically before accepting information as fact. This applies not just to marketing, but to food and diet information, political speech and opinion, and the news media we consume.

I propose that the first and most important step in restoring a sense of control to your life is to *reclaim your diet*. Protesting or going to the occasional political rally is small potatoes compared to eating a diet free of the influence of the food industry.

So cook your own food. Moderate your consumption of fats and sweets. Get to know the facts about product labeling. Start a garden or, if you can't, join a CSA and shop at farmers' markets. *Skip the processed foods and wave the flag of dietary independence.*

Proclivity to Excess

Back to our challenge: Why is dietary moderation/appetite control such a struggle? Why do we have such a deep-seated urge to consume high-fat, sweet, rich foods? The previous section discussed our sensitivity to stimuli as a conditioned response to external influences; this section addresses our hereditary internal cues. We are, in fact, genetically programmed for excess.

The Caveman: Yearning for Excess

From the dawn of our species (approximately 400,000 years ago until about 10,000 years ago) we lived in a feast-or-famine environment. When our tribe came upon a bear or moose we feasted; when we found a grove of ripe berries we ate until our stomachs hurt, storing the excess calories as fat. This was necessary to weather the inevitable times of shortage: a series of unsuccessful hunts or a drought that rendered the landscape barren. A history defined by scarcity favored people with tastes for calorically dense foods and large portions.

Heredity: Benefit and Liability
Genetic mutation is a feature of selective reproduction that allows species to increase their odds of survival. Without mutation, evolution couldn't occur. Individuals with the best genetic variants for their environments survive, reproduce, and pass their traits on to their offspring. Examples include disease resistance, the development of lactose tolerance, the retention of body hair in cold climates, and the protection of melanin-rich dark skin for sunny regions.

It's not only humans who are prone to excess. In the book *Zoobiquity*, cardiologist Barbara Natterson-Horowitz examines the commonalities between animal and human disease, including obesity:

> "Given the chance, many wild fish, reptiles, birds, and mammals will overindulge. [...] "Although we may think of food in the wild as hard to come by, at certain times of the year and under certain conditions, the supply may be unlimited. Seeds spill across fields. Larvae cover sand and vegetation. Eggs lie easily available under every leaf. Bushes fill with berries. Flowers ooze with nectar. And when animals' environments are this abundant, they will gorge. Many stop only when their digestive tracts literally cannot take any more. Tamarin monkeys have been seen to eat so many berries in one sitting that their intestines get overwhelmed and they soon excrete the same whole fruits they recently gobbled down. After gorging on abundant prey, carnivorous fish sometimes start excreting undigested flesh. Big felines, like lions, as a matter of course stuff themselves after a hunt until they can barely move."[3]

The development of agriculture greatly improved our food supply. It also resulted in a booming population, so food supplies remained only moderately more reliable than they were for the hunter-gatherers. It was only in the last few generations that agriculture, via modern plant-breeding wizardry and the use of fossil fuels (nitrogen-based fertilizers, heavy machinery, and irrigation), became so efficient that we now live in a never-ending season of excess. We are as unprepared for this excess as we would be if suddenly all land masses on earth flooded and we became a marine species. We need to learn to swim in rising waters.

The Priest: Managing Excess

"Do not join those who drink too much wine or gorge themselves on meat"
PROVERBS 23:20-21

It is likely that early hunter-gatherers feared, and even worshipped, the natural world. This was a logical perspective for a species that occupied a tenuous middle position in nature's hierarchy. When humans learned to harness nature and create surplus calories, our place in the hierarchy rose. In cultures with monotheistic religion, we swapped a nature-based spirituality for worshipping a divine image similar to ourselves.

Our power expanded rapidly to encompass more than just food production. We restructured ecosystems on a grand scale, created formidable structures, and developed powerful weapons. We then needed to manage our concomitant tendencies to consume in excess and to inflict violence. Religious texts such as the Bible and the Koran gave many societies a framework for the new world; common themes and concepts were how to mediate conflict and how to handle large inequities in wealth. Texts such as these also share a strong emphasis on limiting impulses and contemplating the consequences of selfish actions, all of which made them the logical foundations for early legal systems.

The impact of excess and the need for restraint have also been central questions addressed by philosophers such as Plato and Confucius, religious figures outside the monotheistic tradition such as the Buddha, and contemporary neuroscientists. Psychologist Jonathan Haidt, citing the various beliefs about the conflict inherent in the human condition, describes the mind as an "elephant" of automatic desires and impulses atop which conscious intention is an ineffectual "rider."[4]

Much of the raison d'être for societal institutions is their role as elephant tamers. While government, academia, and religion have had some success in that role—we don't live in a dystopian world of violence, chaos, depravity, and crime—institutions have failed society when it comes to health, and in particular, the obesity crisis.

Conditioning to Excess: We Shall Overcome

Zoobiquity pointed out that our attitude toward calories is not substantially different from that of our fellow animals. As we look back at our grandfathers' generation and wonder what made them so fond of cigarettes, one day our grandchildren will look back and smugly wonder, "How could people have so enthusiastically weakened their bodies with soda, fried food, and ice cream?"

Our ancestors recognized the necessity of controlling the baser impulses inherent in the human psyche and developed moral codes. We are at an analogous evolutionary crossroads in our relationship with diet. This is our moment to forge a new code of behavior, to upgrade our approach. We can work to counter our instinctive urge to indulge. We can choose the lasting value that lies in restraint.

The Way Ahead

As any dieter knows, there are many ways to lose weight; it's harder to find ways to keep it off. Here we'll explore some of the more effective, sustainable techniques.

1 **Health clinic consultation** with a registered dietitian. You can expect sound nutritional advice based on an analysis of your medical history. This technique generally works, but since the time you're investing in behavior change techniques is limited, weight loss comes about slowly. It's also easy for patients to slip back into old habits.

2 **Outpatient programs** run by hospitals and health clinics. Expanding on the first option, these programs offer a mix of private and group consultations that typically meet weekly and run for a few months. The duration and the social support yield better and more sustainable results than individual consultations alone.

3 **Weight loss surgery** (gastric bypass, bands, and related variations). While effective, the surgeries are very expensive, have considerable side effects, carry the risk of complications, and still require rigid adherence to a strict diet. This approach is best for those whose health is severely compromised by obesity and, even then, only when all other (sane) approaches have failed.

4 I have found that the *most* effective weight loss solutions are those that isolate us from our habits, our evolutionary instincts, and our indulgent environment. These include **spas, retreats, and weight loss centers:**

- Rancho La Puerta, mentioned in my profile of Cecilia (Chapter 11), counters its clients' sensitivity to stimuli by replacing everyday influences with environmental cues that promote tranquility, creativity, and physical activity. Resorts like Rancho are less focused on diet than on positive behavior change.

- Shane Diet Resorts and Wellspring Weight Loss Camps, where I've worked as staff dietitian, successfully overcome the evolutionary conditioning to excess consumption. At both places weight loss exceeding 20 pounds per month is run of the mill. Shane and Wellspring are nutritional rehab facilities, carefully simulated re-creations of scarcity. In these settings clients are not allowed second servings of protein or starch, but they do get an abundance of fresh fruits and vegetables. Cravings for sweets and fat are not indulged, but clients can satisfy their appetite with low-calorie, high-volume whole foods.[5] The generous quantities of fruits and vegetables help dieters fight their cravings, which, inevitably, subside over a few weeks.

Our inner elephant's appetite is often tamed with this kind of controlled scarcity or medical deprivation: taking in fewer calories than we need and greatly increasing our physical activity. Other effective tools offered in these settings:

- **Behavioral therapy,** during which participants learn stress management and how to cope with their feelings about food and other life challenges.

- **Nutrition and culinary education,** to teach the science and practice of diet.

- Sports and other types of **physical activity,** which build confidence and burn calories while decreasing stress.

There are many high-quality programs. Make certain to look for options with a registered dietitian, qualified mental health professionals,[6] and certified personal trainers on staff, along with the three tools identified above.

Red Flags

Avoid diet programs that:

1 Promote rapid weight loss in a way that sounds too good to be true: *"Lose 20 pounds in 10 days!"*

2 Use extreme or fad diets (raw, juice-only, cleanses, detoxes, and fasts)

3 Feature grueling exercise regimens (boot camps and other military-inspired workouts)

4 Employ staff with quickie certifications (like "certified nutrition coach" or "holistic life therapist") from unaccredited schools

5 Prey on cynicism about mainstream medicine: *"We have the cure that 'They' don't want you to know about!"*

6 Exploit positive associations with other causes: environmental, humanitarian, or religious/spiritual*

7 Promote the use of proprietary supplements and superfoods

* *Organic food, Buddhist theology, and solar-powered cottages are wonderful, but they shouldn't be used to disguise a flawed program.*

The problem with some programs is not that the diets, workouts, or supplements are inherently unhealthy. Following a super-strict diet and engaging in intense workouts can help you look and feel great. **The problem is a lack of sustainability.** For most people, eating highly restrictive diets and spending hours per day doing yoga, weight training, hiking, or swimming is just not realistic. When a routine isn't sustainable, excess weight returns, often with feelings of guilt, shame, and failure. These experiences can prompt you to completely abandon your health goals ("It's just too hard!") or trigger even more dangerous cycles of deprivation followed by indulgence: periods of intense workouts and over-the-top dieting followed by periods of sedentary behavior and unhealthy eating. In some cases this behavior leads to full-blown eating disorders: orthorexia, bulimia, and anorexia.

NOTES

1 Martin Lindstrom, *Buyology: Truth and Lies About Why We Buy* (New York: Doubleday, 2008), 49-50, 79-80.

2 Lindstrom, *Brandwashed: Tricks Companies Use to Manipulate Our Minds and Persuade Us to Buy* (New York: Crown Business, 2010), 63-64.

3 Barbara Natterson-Horowitz, *Zoobiquity: The Astonishing Connection Between Human and Animal Health* (New York: Random House, 2012), 135-136.

4 Jonathan Haidt is a psychology professor at New York University. He researches morality and is the author of *The Happiness Hypothesis* and *The Righteous Mind: Why Good People are Divided by Politics and Religion.*

5 Wellspring's diet was 70% carbohydrate, 20% protein, 10% fat; Shane's was 60% carbohydrate, 20% protein, 20% fat.

6 Look for these qualifications: masters in social work (MSW), marriage and family therapist (MFT), and/or licensed master social worker (LMSW).

CHAPTER 13

The Last Refuge of the Hedonist

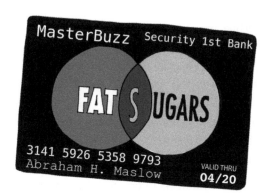

When your needs aren't being met... there's MasterBuzz*

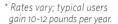

* Rates vary; typical users gain 10-12 pounds per year.

CAN YOU IMAGINE A THANKSGIVING DINNER of celery sticks, rice, and split peas or a wedding banquet of mineral water, crackers, and hummus? Would you usher in the new year with friends by raising a glass of milk at midnight? Part of what makes our celebrations memorable is the high that indulgence offers, whether it comes in the form of too many calories or by means of mind-altering substances.

The National Buzz

Cheers! ¡Salud! Santé! Na zdorov'ya! Ege'szse'gedre! L'chaim!

Psychologist Abraham Maslow called pleasure an evolutionarily motivator, noting that it's hard-wired—we continue behavior that brings us pleasure, and avoid that which does not. As discussed in Chapter 10, most cultures have customs that define appropriate times for excess, such as religious events and rites of passage. It follows that there are also rules and rituals for the appropriate use of intoxicants. Many Middle Eastern and African cultures ban alcohol but allow hookah smoking and the use of the stimulant khat. The indigenous people of the Andes chew coca leaves as a mild stimulant, to ameliorate altitude sickness, and to help ward off cold and hunger. In Pacific Island cultures the herb kava is widely used in social settings for its sedative, euphoric, and mildly psychoactive effects. In parts of India and Southeast

Asia, chewing the stimulant betel nut is as common a social ritual as coffee drinking is in the United States.

Cyclical Taboos: the USA and Its Contradictions

In the United States, alcohol was established early on as our principal—though not only—sanctioned vice.

> "While precise consumption figures are lacking, informed estimates suggest that by the 1790s an average American over 15 years old drank just under six gallons of absolute alcohol each year. That represented some thirty-four gallons of beer and cider (about 3.4 gallons of absolute alcohol), slightly over five gallons of distilled liquors (2.3 gallons of absolute alcohol), and under a gallon of wine (possibly .10 gallons absolute). Because this is an average figure... the level of consumption probably was much higher for actual drinkers."[1]

To put these numbers in perspective, they are well over double the amount of current alcohol consumption.

The liberal attitude toward intoxication established by our founders continued unabated for about 150 years until Prohibition (1920–1933), a not-so-dry minute in our national happy hour. Pervasive drinking in violation of the law was one of the reasons for Prohibition's repeal, and the legal partying quickly resumed.

The 1950s, '60s, and '70s stand out as particularly indulgent times, with high rates of cigarette smoking and spirited exploration of drugs, both legal and illegal. Among the legal drugs, speed (mostly amphetamines in the form of widely prescribed diet pills) was consumed by millions across a diverse spectrum of society.[2] Alcohol, too: My father told stories of his time as a young reporter in Washington, D.C., during the heyday of print journalism, the 1960s and '70s. Then, daytime meetings typically included alcohol, the better to loosen the lips of reporters' sources: carefully scripted lawyers, politicians, lobbyists, and businessmen. Reporters stumbling in from long, boozy lunches were a regular sight in the newsroom. The drunken fellows would sleep away the afternoon on an office couch, then stay at work until late evening, banging away on their typewriters until an article was finished.

The 1980s brought sweeping changes. A moral righteousness, an echo of Prohibition, was on the rise. Daytime drinking as a part of work culture was no longer tolerated. A growing recognition of the seriousness and public health consequences of alcoholism, the toxicity of tobacco, and the addictive quality of many drugs gave rise to movements such as Mothers Against Drunk Driving (MADD), anti-smoking campaigns, and First Lady Nancy Reagan's "Just Say No" antidrug awareness program. In a signal shift toward a more restrictive society, we began to reject the culture of hedonism.

Alcohol use in the U.S. has declined steadily since 1980 — from 2.76 gallons of pure ethanol to 2.32 gallons in 2008,[3] a decrease of 16 percent in 28 years. The trends in tobacco and coffee use are similar; both peaked near the middle of the 20th century and have declined steadily since.

Food's Still Legal, Right?

In the 1980s, as American attitudes towards intoxication grew stricter and tolerance of drinking and smoking waned, food became the last refuge of the hedonist. The three-martini lunch (or beers in the break room) became the midday free-for-all, with fried chicken, subs, ribs, potato salad, chips, cake, candy, coffee, juices, and sodas. The all-you-can-eat buffet continued on the weekend, where being the "hostess with the mostest" no longer referred to having a fully stocked liquor cabinet or hand-rolled cigars, but rather to serving an extensive array of calorically rich party foods. Rich food seemed so innocent in comparison to past excesses. We added a further layer of decadence with the advent of supersized portions in the late 1980s. It is no coincidence that the Reagan era marks the tipping point of our free fall into obesity.

We are seeing the repercussions of this excess today. Over the past 30 years obesity rates in the United States have doubled in children and quadrupled in adolescents.[4] Since 1980 the worldwide prevalence of diabetes, heart disease, and high blood pressure has more than doubled.[5] Just as the careless use of intoxicants came under scrutiny, we are becoming aware that we can't easily live with the consequences of high-calorie diets.

Man Cannot Live by Bread Alone

Power abhors a vacuum, and apparently so does a good buzz. As society searches for less-fattening escapes, the two emerging candidates look to be pharmaceutical drugs and marijuana.

According to the Centers for Disease Control, 48.7 percent of all adult Americans use at least one prescription drug a month.[6] A similar study by the Mayo Clinic found that the number is almost 70 percent.[7] Although not all of these drugs affect our mental state, many do. While antidepressants, antianxiety meds, sedatives, and psychoactive drugs come quickly to mind, there are many other medications that affect mood: hormone replacement drugs, certain oral contraceptives, attention disorder medications, painkillers (particularly opiate-based painkillers such as OxyContin), medications to control blood sugar, steroids, and the stimulants used to control heart and lung diseases.

Unlike drugs or alcohol used to celebrate at a weekend party or to give a concentration boost the night before an exam, many pharmaceuticals stay in our bloodstream for prolonged periods. Some are designed to work around the clock, meaning that our perception of reality is altered on a long-term basis.

I don't recommend changing your drug regimen without consulting your physician, but it's worthwhile to consider how your medications affect your state of mind.

A modest proposal: When government experts assess the potential for national disaster (nuclear meltdown, terrorist attack) they should also consider what might happen if pharmaceutical manufacturers were unable to deliver their product.

Though many pharmaceutical drugs have strong side effects, including weight gain, they have the perception of being calorie free, the advantage of being discreet, and the assurance that comes with a medical endorsement. The growing use of pharmaceuticals that affect brain activity has likely been a factor in the increasingly successful efforts to legalize marijuana. If one person treats anxiety with a strong pharmaceutical drug and another uses marijuana, is it reasonable that the second deserves a prison sentence? As our taboos shift we realize that the old way of thinking—"my medication is okay, yours is immoral or unhealthy"—is too simple.

It appears that we're undergoing another metamorphosis: turning away from 30-plus years of a "thou-shalt-not" temperament toward a more tolerant mindset that has its own flaws. Every buzz now comes wrapped up with an authority figure's permission slip. You want to smoke marijuana or take a pill to alleviate anxiety? Drink a few cups of coffee or glasses of wine every day? Eat chocolate every night and cook every meal with a huge splash of olive oil? Regardless of your choice, *someone* will assure you it's a healthy decision.

....

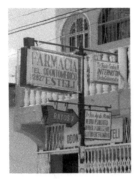

Latin America is the fastest-growing pharmaceutical market in the world.[8] You can't go more than a few blocks in any Nicaraguan town without seeing a pharmacy. Among many reasons for the boom: increasing wealth (the ability to purchase drugs); the rapid rise in disease brought about by changing diets and lifestyles; the elevated status of Western medicine (as opposed to traditional healers); and a greater awareness that drugs are available not just to treat typical diseases (diabetes, malaria), but also for a myriad of conditions such as depression, anxiety, and insomnia. *(Esteli)*

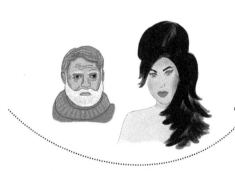

On the other end of the spectrum, the sobriety of Mother Teresa and the Dalai Lama helped them have long, full lives of wisdom and charity.

Ernest Hemingway and Amy Winehouse are examples of medicating to excess. While their substance use may have contributed to their artistic brilliance it also shortened their lives.

Between these extremes the degree of sobriety becomes less clear, especially in the 21st century. Where do legally prescribed and appropriately used pharmaceuticals fit in? Medical marijuana? How about rich food and overeating?

Sobriety, like health, exists on a continuum. Most of us don't seem to be willing to be sober one hundred percent of the time. It's not what you choose to alter your reality that's important; instead, what's important is that you *consider where you stand on the spectrum of sobriety.* Do what you like, but don't fool yourself.

Defining Sobriety

Sobriety once meant that you could touch your finger to your nose and walk in a straight line while explaining to the police officer that you were making a midnight trip to the convenience store, which you were astonished to notice was next door to a bar. Before the onslaught of modern foods, and drugs both legal and illegal, sobriety was simple to define. You were either staggering or not. Now the police and judicial system are grappling with how to legally define drivers sleepily swerving on Ambien hangovers, zombie-fied from painkillers, or so amped up on stimulants that they think a city street is a freeway.

Dietary Intoxication

Food, like air and water, can't be considered addictive because it is essential to life. Nonetheless, eating changes your state of mind because the very act of eating (regardless of the type of food) is of such primal importance that it takes precedence over other drives. Emotion is rooted in matters of survival such as fear (of starvation, of predators) and contentment (like the feeling that comes with safety or a full stomach).

Calorically dense foods are the exception. They share at least two characteristics with intoxicants: they are not essential to life and they can be habit forming. The effects of eating rich foods follow a pattern similar to drug use: dietary excess artificially elevates mood. The flip side — the crash — has an even greater sway on sobriety. As that external kick fades we are left with symptoms like fatigue, crankiness, fragility, frustration, and brain fog. In these vulnerable moments we are tempted to reach for a cup of coffee, a pastry, a handful of nuts, or some other treat to make us feel better. These are perfect conditions for the development of a vicious cycle.

There's another parallel to examine. Law enforcement is not the only entity to notice that there are a diverse range of intoxicants with an equally diverse sway on our judgment. When we think about the attraction of rich food, we should remind ourselves that an appeal to appetite is in itself a form of behavior manipulation. Why do so many retail establishments — car dealerships, banks, investment offices, art galleries, luxury clothing stores — offer their customers free food and drink? Sales managers are keen students of human behavior; they understand that decision making is affected by how full or empty our stomachs are. Those tempting treats (and the implication of the seller's generosity) can give nervous customers the extra push they need to make a major purchase, loan, or investment.

For a historical perspective on the influence of calorie-rich food we can look at what happened to other cultures when they were introduced to powerful substances.

By the time Europeans made contact and began actively trading goods (including distilled spirits) with the Americas, they had been drinking alcohol for thousands of years. Their bodies adapted over generations to produce enzymes that metabolize alcohol rapidly. Indigenous Americans, having limited exposure to alcohol (largely in less-potent forms), had far fewer enzymes to metabolize it. They became inebriated faster and developed addictions at a much higher rate than Europeans. Additionally, while indigenous Americans were relatively naïve to alcohol's power, most Europeans had known, or at least heard, of someone's life ruined by alcohol. They grew up in cultures full of warnings, fables, and stories that explained its special properties. Vulnerable on both the cultural and biological fronts, indigenous Americans suffered greatly (and continue to suffer) from excess alcohol consumption.

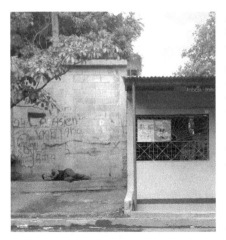

Anesthetize your present, mortgage your future.

When I left for work at 8:00 AM, I often saw this fellow passed out by the wall, a block from my house. When I returned in the early evening he would still be there, in the same position. Most neighborhoods in Managua have a few dedicated drunks. While combating alcoholism is one of the top priorities for Nicaragua's Ministry of Health, on a local level alcoholics are viewed with compassion and are generally accepted as just another element of the community. (*Managua*)

We are in a similar situation with calorie-rich foods. We can't metabolize the large quantities of sugars and fat at the rate we consume them. We are naïve to their effects—or we widely underestimate them—and we are developing addictions. Given a few thousand years our genes might mutate just enough to allow us to handle caloric density and maintain a normal weight.

But we can't wait for natural selection (a biological solution). It's up to us to develop a cultural solution. While previous campaigns against excess—Prohibition and the fantastically expensive, multidecade "war on drugs"—were ineffective, today we have the opportunity to broker a dietary treaty instead of launching another war. We can chart a more sustainable course, including vigorous nutrition education in schools, stronger government regulation, and recognition of the value of periodic, measured breaks from sobriety.

Whether it is eating cake on your birthday, drinking champagne on New Year's Eve, or ringing in the harvest with piles of roasted pig meat, marking special occasions with excess is a universal part of human culture. A cradle-to-grave sober existence is unnatural, not to mention unrealistic. Additionally, there are many well-studied benefits to (occasional) altered states, including heightened creativity and an increase in empathy that strengthens social ties. You must decide what is healthy for you: perhaps this means you are disciplined six days a week and you have a Sabbath on the seventh day, when you gather with family and friends and eat liberally. Perhaps it means coffee and pastries on Saturday morning, beers with Sunday football...

...or the once-a decade trip to Peru.

The Peruvian Solution

In 2011 I had the opportunity to learn about shamanism—a subject that had long fascinated me—during a four-month stay in Peru. Prior to Western influence, the indigenous people of Peru didn't have the option of medicating their troubles with pharmaceutical drugs, alcohol, or processed food. One of the traditional medicines of the region was (and still is) ayahuasca. Like the other substances discussed in this chapter, ayahuasca removes one from sobriety and can be misused. However, with the proper guidance it has therapeutic benefits. Peruvian shamans are famous for the phyto-spiritual "surgery" they facilitate with their patients. Using ayahuasca, a strong hallucinogen, they guide participants on an inner journey with common goals including uncovering insights into problems and healing both physical and emotional traumas. As befits a book focused on sobriety, I will skip the sexy discussion on the controversial psychedelic aspect of the custom and instead explore the role diet plays in the process.

I interviewed several shamans, all of whom strongly recommend a period of dietary cleansing from several weeks to several months prior to taking ayahuasca. The belief is that a strict regime prepares one for the vigors of the powerful visions and emotions that await. Shamans call this *la dieta*, the diet. Typical restrictions include salt, sugar, chocolate, spices, and chiles; fats and oils; canned and processed food; red meat and pork; vinegar; caffeine, stimulants, and alcohol; and all recreational drugs and pharmaceuticals.

One particularly memorable visit I made was to a shaman in the small mountain village of Taray, a few hours east of the famous ruins of Machu Picchu. We discussed many things, including the rise of tourism, the modernization of Peru, and his work, but he was especially passionate on the subject of diet. Here is an excerpt from our conversation:

Why is it important to follow the diet prior to the ayahuasca ceremony?
The experience of ayahuasca starts with the knowledge gained during cleansing. The participant arrives to the session with an already modified state of consciousness.

How can following a strict diet affect consciousness?
Every food has a message; some are stronger than others. Following the diet cleanses the mind from conflicting messages. Ayahuasca is a *plantamaestra*, a professor plant; it has a great deal to teach. If your body has been influenced by strong foods then it can't give itself completely to the ayahuasca.

How can diet impede the experience?

Sugar, caffeine, flesh, and heavy foods [fats] modify consciousness. They have a strong influence. The ayahuasca plant is jealous over the power they have.

How can a plant be jealous?

The body isn't free and independent with those foods exerting their control. The healing and revelatory effects of ayahuasca work much better if the body is free.

Is there a physical reaction as well, or are you only talking about the effect on the mind?

It is difficult to separate the effects, but yes, those who follow the diet don't throw up as much, get sick, or feel weak. In general, they feel stronger. The experience goes more smoothly for them.

Outside of diet, what recommendations are there for altering one's lifestyle prior to working with ayahuasca?

The goal is to take away outside influences as much as possible. One should avoid overexposure to rain, sun, smoke, fire, polluted air, and foul odors. One must abstain from sexual activities for at least two weeks, but longer is better. Also, interacting with people who are strongly pessimistic or sick should be avoided.

Why are these practices important?

We weaken the power of our material desires and the cultural influences that separate us from nature. In this way we can be more open to guidance and power from the plant world, from ayahuasca.

Shamans have a firm belief that diet affects consciousness. They single out as having undue influence many of the foods we crave: sweets, salty snacks, rich and heavy foods, alcohol, and coffee. As a dietitian I couldn't help appreciating the respect they had for the transformative power of diet. It also caused me to speculate whether we North Americans can channel our desire for altered states in a safe, ritual manner.

NOTES

1 Mark Edward Lender, *Drinking In America: A History* (New York: Free Press, 1987), 14.

2 Nicolas Rasmussen, "America's First Amphetamine Epidemic 1929–1971: A Quantitative and Qualitative Retrospective With Implications for the Present." *Am J Public Health* 98 (June 2008): 974–985.

3 Robin LaVallee et al., *Apparent Per Capita Alcohol Consumption: National, State, and Regional Trends, 1977–2012*. U.S. Department of Health and Human Services, 2014.

4 *Childhood Obesity: CDC Childhood Obesity Prevention Fact Sheet, 2015*, (Atlanta, GA: Division of Population Health, National Center for Chronic Disease Prevention and Health Promotion).

5 Statistics on diabetes rates from "Worldwide trends in diabetes since 1980: a pooled analysis of 751 population-based studies with 4.4 million participants." *The Lancet* 387 (April 6, 2016): 1513–30.

6 National Center for Health Statistics. *Health, United States, 2015: With Special Feature on Racial and Ethnic Health Disparities*, (Hyattsville, MD: U.S. Department of Health and Human Services, 2016), 271–272.

7 Zhong et al., "Age and Sex Patterns of Drug Prescribing in a Defined American Population." *Mayo Clinic Proceedings* 88 (July 2013): 697–707.

8 John Price, "Latin America's Booming Pharma Industry Is A Local Affair," *Latin Trade*, October 8, 2013.

CHAPTER 14

The Stockholm Syndrome

"I came in contact with those who were regarded as pillars of vegetarianism, and began my own experiments in dietetics. I stopped taking the sweets and condiments I had got from home. The mind having taken a different turn, the fondness for condiments wore away, and I now relished the boiled spinach which in Richmond tasted insipid, cooked without condiments. Many such experiments taught me that the real seat of taste was not of the tongue but the mind."[1]

MAHATMA GANDHI

IN THE GRASSY PLAINS OF THE HUNGARIAN COUNTRYSIDE there once lived a farmer who raised goats, sheep, and chickens. The farmer was an anxious fellow who had long suffered from being a light sleeper. One morning, after a particularly fitful night, he sought his rabbi's advice. The rabbi suggested that he bring a few chickens to stay inside the house. The farmer did as told. The next day he returned to the rabbi, complaining that the chickens' squawking made it even harder for him to sleep. The rabbi replied that he must bring a few goats into the house. Despite his doubts, the pious farmer did as told. This cycle continued for a week, with the rabbi answering the increasingly weary farmer's complaints with stern instructions that more animals were to be brought inside. Finally, with half of the farm sleeping under the same roof, the rabbi relented and told the farmer that it was time to send all the animals from his house. The farmer returned to the rabbi the following day. Cheerful and well rested, he proclaimed that he had never known such peace.

A few centuries later the farmer's descendant walks into a grocery store on a scorching summer day. The moment she steps inside a wave of crisp air washes over her, and she relishes the refreshing coolness. Ten minutes later, as she finishes paying for her handful of items, she no longer notices the air conditioning. As she exits the store an intoxicating whiff of roasting coffee beans beckons her into an adjacent coffee shop. She buys a coffee and stirs in a teaspoon of sugar. By the time she sips the last drop, her nose no longer acknowledges the aroma that had enticed her only minutes before. On her way out she realizes she forgot to buy coffee at the grocery store, so she purchases two pounds of coffee beans in a burlap bag. Noting the bag's barbell-like heft in her grip, she playfully performs a few bicep curls. She stuffs the bag into her already full backpack, where it squeezes in with the groceries, a book, and a laptop. As she strolls out of the store her backpack does not feel noticeably heavier.

Was the farmhouse ever quiet?
Was the temperature inside the grocery store perfect?
Does a teaspoon of sugar make coffee sweet?
Was the bag of beans heavy?

There are no absolute answers. The farmhouse seemed quieter once the animals left. The air in the store was cool in contrast to the air outside. If you rarely have sweets, your coffee will taste sweet with a small amount of sugar, but if you eat sweets regularly, you will desire another teaspoon or even two. A weight that feels substantial in your hand can be imperceptible when added to an already heavy backpack. Our senses quickly acclimate to each new environment, and while they are excellent at assessing comparative values, they are not designed for determining absolutes.

When we remove all the richest and sweetest tastes from our diet, we are making use of the architecture of our senses. One can think of calorie-dense foods as heavy drapes. Their removal invites the sunshine in, allowing us to evaluate the food we do eat in a far more flattering light. Regardless of which diet we follow our taste buds will adapt, so it makes sense to train them to adapt to a diet that gives us the body and the health we desire.

A Quick Experiment
Take a bite of a sweet fruit, chew it, and enjoy the flavor. Next, take a bite of a dessert (candy, ice cream, or pastry). Try the fruit again — you'll find that it no longer tastes as sweet.

In 1973 a group of Swedes were held hostage for six days in a vault during a bank robbery. Over those six days the hostages' fear and anger subsided and they grew attached to their captors. Psychologists believe that sympathizing with one's oppressors is common, even predictable; they coined the term the **Stockholm syndrome** to define the process. This syndrome can develop in a variety of unhealthy relationships, including child abuse, spousal abuse, and cult member/leader relationships.

When it comes to unhealthy diets we exhibit behavior similar to the Stockholm syndrome, becoming acclimated to, and held captive by, a diet that is harming us.

Choose carefully...

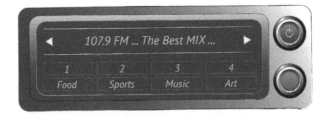

What You Tune Into Tunes You

Prior to the 20th century humans adapted to the fairly narrow diets available in their local regions. Now, many of us have access to a wide array of foods. Our diets can be oriented toward **need** (what a healthy body requires) or **desire** (the craving for a hedonic experience). Because we're faced with so many choices, it is useful to consider what happens when we narrow our focus or refocus our senses altogether.

Our appreciation for anything is proportional to the degree we dedicate our senses to it. Consider food festivals (e.g., the Southwest Chocolate and Coffee Fest, the Blue Ribbon Bacon Festival, and the American Royal World Series of Barbecue). Typically these skip dietary staples and low-calorie foods (currently there is no Celebrity Celery Crunchfest) and focus on hedonic foods like cheese, chocolate, seafood, and meat. In addition to celebrating calorie-dense delights, these gatherings exist so that those who have taken the time to develop highly tuned palates can discuss, appreciate, and debate the variations in flavor that would otherwise go unappreciated by untrained tongues.

The quintessential example of the tuned palate is the wine connoisseur. Perhaps you've chatted with one at a party. He or she might comment that the Cabernet Sauvignon you're both drinking has a velvety oak flavor with grippy tannins. You might have sensed a mild woody flavor, so you nod in polite agreement—though you hadn't noticed a velvety texture and, while you've heard of tannins, you have no idea how to recognize them or what a "grippy" tannin is.

We don't become experts on any food or drink if we consume it only a few times a month. A sommelier drinks wine—or at least tastes it—daily. This practice develops taste buds that, with a few sips, can accurately determine the type of grapes that compose a wine, how well the wine has aged, the type of vessel it was aged in, the region it comes from, and possibly the vintage. An experienced sommelier matches a trained palate to a patient mind that has invested time in acquiring knowledge of the wine-making process: fermenting techniques, harvest times, climates, and soils.

The investment of time required to become a discerning consumer of a particular alcoholic beverage or certain calorie-rich foods is one example of fine-tuning the senses. For those with no weight problems such interests can constitute an enriching hobby. The rest of us might consider tuning our senses to another frequency. For instance, we could use that time to become more appreciative of or skilled in music, art, language, science, architecture, literature, film, or sport. If we do focus on food, at least we should focus on the foods that will allow us to reach our optimum health and weight.

Food Sobriety is an example of a goal-oriented approach to diet. It also involves training the palate. When the Amazon River of modern cuisine is narrowed to a stream of cyclical flavors, your taste buds will discern the distinctions between pinto and kidney beans, yellow-dent corn and classic sweet corn, the butternut and the acorn squash. A diet that at first seems pedestrian grows increasingly satisfying when you can detect subtle differences.

Tuning the Ear

The focus inherent in fine-tuning works with all our senses, not only our sense of taste. I first made this connection when, as an undergraduate, I took several music theory classes. In the ear-training parts of these classes, our professor gave us exercises in which we listened to two notes and tried to identity the interval — the amount of space between the notes. (A "fifth," for instance, is two notes that are five notes apart.) At first I found this exercise frustrating; the various intervals blurred together. In particular, fourths and fifths sounded the same to me, and I often confused thirds and sixths.

Our professor, who had a side interest in neuroscience, explained that the human brain in "learning mode" acts like a computer dedicating increasing amounts of its hard drive to a project. He described how our brains would grow additional neurons in proportion to the hours we spent doing our ear-training tutorials. In response to music study the brain expands the aural neural network to finely tune the sense of hearing, in much the same way lifting weights increases muscle size. He was right — within a few weeks we could easily recognize all the intervals, and by midsemester we were rapidly identifying long strings of notes. By finals we were able to transcribe the entire melodic and harmonic structure of long compositions.

A musician expands aural neural networks, a painter expands visual ones, and a foodie expands those connected to the sense of taste. *Where do you want to focus?*

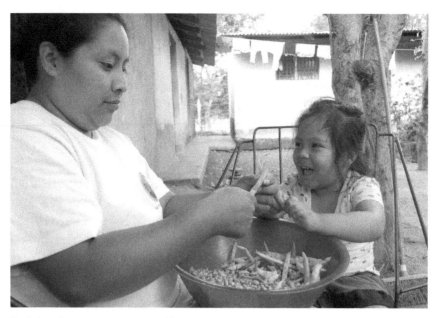

Training the next generation of bean connoisseurs. Lourdes is teaching her grand-daughter, Gabriella, how to shell beans. Most of Lourdes' harvest will be spread on tarps to dry under the sun. Dried beans can be stored and eaten year round. Like most bean farmers, Lourdes also enthusiastically sets aside a small part of her harvest without drying. *Frijoles nuevos* (new beans) stay fresh for only a few weeks, cook in half the time of regular dried beans and, as any bean connoisseur knows, have the most delicious flavor: succulent and bright, with a touch of fruitlike light-ness. Nicaraguans enjoy the new beans when they are available — for a few weeks after the biannual harvests. *(El Jicaro)*

Tuning Up the Youth

The summer of 2010 was the first of my summers with the weight loss company Wellspring Camps. I collaborated with our host, the University of California at San Diego, to redesign their cafeteria menu. We came up with a two-week cyclical menu — what the clients ate on June 15th was the same as what they'd have on June 30th. During the first few weeks of camp, I got many complaints. A curly-headed teenage camper, Nestor, complained that the lasagna "looked and tasted exactly like cardboard." He clearly wasn't used to the flavor of whole-wheat pasta, low-fat cheese, and extra-lean ground turkey. Tabatha, a tall, feisty, college-age blonde with a wild sense of humor, bitterly protested the chicken stir-fry: "The proportions are all wrong, I want meat, meat, meat! After I am done sorting out all the veggies I despise, I have only enough food to feed a pigeon." I never argued with the campers, but listened attentively and assured them I'd see what I could do to improve the food.

Two weeks later, Nestor dropped by the dinner table to congratulate me on the lasagna. "Hey, Dan, you are a magician. You turned cardboard into real lasagna. Thanks for fixing the recipe." A few days later it was Tabatha's turn. "Dan, my man! You are *rocking* the kitchen these days. The stir-fry is delicious; I'm stuffed!" Soon enough I was hearing these 180-degree reversals every day. I had to put my hand over my mouth to cover my devious smile because the truth was that I had done nothing to deserve their praise.

UCSD had a large commercial kitchen that ordered food from a nationwide distributor. Neither the recipes nor the ingredients ever varied: the brand of pasta, the canned tomatoes, the frozen, pre-marinated chicken breasts. The only flexible element in the equation was the taste buds of the campers. By the end of the summer I let the campers in on the truth and we shared a few laughs about the situation, though it no longer mattered much to them. They learned a far more exciting secret: they could thrive despite being limited to simple, low-calorie food. Steak and french fries had been replaced by the confidence of a strengthening body and the warmth of new friendships.

First Adopters and Sensory Balance

"Nothing in the world is worth having or worth doing unless it means effort, pain, difficulty.... I have never in my life envied a human being who led an easy life. I have envied a great many people who led difficult lives and led them well."
THEODORE ROOSEVELT

In Jonathan Swift's classic *Gulliver's Travels,* the protagonist finds himself marooned on an island of talking horses where he survives on the simplest of foods.

> "The horse immediately ordered a white mare servant of his family to bring me a good quantity of oats in a sort of wooden tray. These I heated before the fire, as well as I could, and rubbed them till the husks came off, which I made a shift to winnow from the grain. I ground and beat them between two stones; then took water, and made them into a paste or cake, which I toasted at the fire and ate warm with milk. It was at first a very insipid diet, though common enough in many parts of Europe, but grew tolerable by time; and having been often reduced to hard fare in my life, this was not the first experiment I had made how easily nature is satisfied."[2]

The experience of **thriving despite a limited menu** is why my patients who most readily adopted the Food Sobriety philosophy often came from backgrounds that included a Gulliver-esque chapter involving isolation: missionaries, military veterans, Peace Corps volunteers, sailors, immigrants, campers, backpackers, fishermen, hunters, and many varieties of scientists involved in field research. All of these people faced times when their food choice was limited. Several weeks into their adventure they had the "ah-ha" moment: when the biscuits, beef jerky, and freeze-dried vegetables became tasty or when the instant mashed potatoes and powdered milk transformed from barely tolerable to enjoyable.

This unique group not only had been isolated from making bad food choices but also often had experienced stimulating environments that engaged the senses: the great outdoors, travel, new cultures, danger, foreign languages, the thrill of learning and living in the moment, and, perhaps most importantly, a meaningful purpose or goal. (When you're pulling a 25-pound salmon out of a rushing river or helping a community build a school, you don't need an artisanal maple-glazed almond-oat scone to remind you how special life is.)

While most of us aren't fortunate enough to lead lives consistently brimming with meaning and constructive challenges, we can probably relate to some of those vivid experiences, for instance, in everything that nature has to offer. We all love to see leaves fall in autumn, snowflakes float down in winter, and flowers bloom in spring. But the experience is not just visual. Each season, even each day, has distinctive sights, smells, textures, sounds, and tastes. Imagine when you walked barefoot and felt every change beneath your feet: hot sand; wet moss; rough stone; a grassy meadow.

We have a finite ability to take in sensory stimulation. When one sense gets more input, another gets less. An extreme example is that those who lose a sense, such as the blind, find that another sense grows much more powerful (à la the exceptionally talented blind musicians who have perfect pitch). Cultures, like people, also have distinctive sensory priorities. Some cultures are more visual and focus on elaborate textiles, fashion/personal ornamentation, murals, paintings, and architecture. In Nicaragua, hearing is the dominant sense, though it overlaps with the sense of touch, since dancing and music are so closely intertwined. In the USA, the most diverse, abundant, and hedonistic food supply on earth has had a profound sway on our sensory priorities.

Sensory Budgets of Cultures

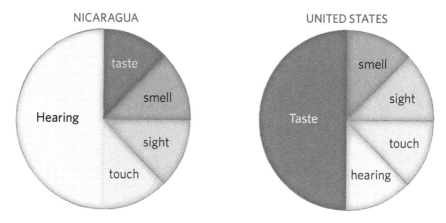

NICARAGUA

UNITED STATES

What does *your* sensory budget look like?

Sight, smell, touch, hearing, and taste exist in balance. The earth, subjugated by modernity, can no longer offer us its full cornucopia of sounds, sights, textures, smells, and (natural) tastes. We spend our lives increasingly isolated from nature: few of us engage in spring planting, summer weeding, and fall hunting. Even so, because we evolved in the natural world, we still crave change in our stimuli. We instinctively feel more at ease if we bear witness to growth, softening, ripening, and decay in the world, but we're surrounded by man-made constructs—office buildings, homes, and city streets—designed to resist the effects of nature. A side effect of modern life is that our senses are understimulated; this creates an urge to make up for the sensory deficiency, and the easiest way to close the gap is with our taste buds.

Over the past century the culture in the United States has shifted toward this comfortable, seductive focus on taste. In Nicaragua, even though the diet is rapidly modernizing and the culture is becoming more taste oriented, the aural sense still dominates. Music is everywhere. It pours from churches, homes, businesses, and street corners. Nicas sing their hearts out without a shred of inhibition—whether secular or religious, in public or in private, on-pitch or wildly off-key. The only feeling more liberating than listening to Nicaraguans sing is joining one of their spontaneous dance parties. They occur frequently, and all ages and skill levels are always encouraged and applauded.

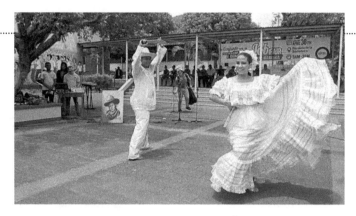

Dancing at UNAN

During my tenure at the National Autonomous University of Nicaragua in Managua I was invited to an end-of-semester party. Because the party was at lunchtime and was only for the fairly small nutrition staff, I was expecting a mellow affair. I showed up at noon surprised to see nearly 100 people gathered in front of a massive professional PA system. A few minutes later Latin music started and the first of three superb dance troupes of students came out. The first troupe performed several indigenous-inspired dances, including the most famous national piece, *El Güegüense,* a satirical drama that tells the story of indigenous people and their early interactions with Spaniards. The second group performed colonial-era courtship dances featuring enormous dresses that looked tremendously uncomfortable in the tropical heat. The third performance ditched almost all clothes and was a sweaty, sexy, modern affair of fast-moving dancers flying back and forth across the stage.

Well, that does it for the dance portion of the party; now we just nibble and chat about micronutrients, right? Hardly. The moment the professional dancers exited, the faculty and their families took over. The next three hours were nonstop dancing. Though every type of Latin music played, there were also surprises: Katy Perry, the Beatles, and Amy Winehouse. Regardless of the musical style everyone danced with the passion of the professionals — exhibiting nearly the same skill — and sang along with the lyrics. I danced with a great-grandmother, a secretary, two professors, and one eight-year-old. All of my partners were much better dancers than I was — I was fortunate that they taught me a few moves. For an American to see such an explosion of dance at a faculty party in the middle of the day (with no alcohol) was an unforgettable reminder that the role of music and dance in Latin culture far surpasses their role in North America.

The "Uncivilized" Perspective

It's not just the adventuresome among us who share a willingness to reconsider diet's place in their lives. Another experience that can complement a successful switch to food sobriety is exposure to the dietary rules prescribed by certain religions—for example, Muslim halal or Jewish kosher laws. These practices habituate their followers to the idea that diet can serve a purpose beyond pleasure, status, or convenience. It can be a means to achieve a goal, whether to show fidelity to a deity or culture or simply to lighten the body. Whatever the rationale, the key is to acknowledge that a meaningful life is attainable despite dietary restrictions and challenges. Meaning can even be found, in some measure, as a result of those voluntary restrictions.

This dietary outlook is still common in a few areas of Latin America, where, because of a combination of isolation, illiteracy, and lack of electricity, there are few outside influences (TV, radio, internet, newspapers, magazines). When I interviewed these more traditional peoples about their diet, the topic often sparked amusement:

> *"Please describe for me your daily diet."*
> "Food, you know, beans and corn."
>
> *"What else?"*
> "What else, what do you mean? It is plenty."
>
> *"I mean do you eat any other foods?"*
> "Vegetables and fruit."
>
> *"What kinds of vegetables and fruit, and how much?"*
> "Whatever is ripe, we eat. We eat till we feel full."
>
> *"How about animal foods, like meat and cheese?"*
> "When we have a party we sometimes are able to get meat and cheese."
>
> *"That is very interesting. Please explain how often these parties occur and how much meat and cheese is eaten?"*
> [Laughter] "Dan, you are a strange man. What does it matter? We take a break from work and sit with our families, and we thank God for whatever there is available to eat and we enjoy it."

Over and over again I noted a lack of focus on food. They thought it was peculiar that I was studying it and found my questions almost hilariously irrelevant: "Here comes the gringo with the food obsession." Traditional people speak a different language around food. There is no negativity, neurosis, or attempt to proclaim status.

Another example of this perspective comes from the work of Daniel Everett, a linguist who spent years in the remote Amazon with the Pirahã, an isolated tribe.

> "One reason I find Pirahã views of food interesting is that the subject seems less important in some sense to them than it is in my own culture. Obviously they have to eat to live. And they enjoy eating. Whenever there is food available in the village, they eat it all. But life is so full of priorities for all of us, and food is ranked differently by different people and different societies. The Pirahãs have talked to me about why they don't hunt or fish some days when they are hungry. Instead, they might play tag or play with my wheelbarrow, or lie around and talk. 'Why aren't you fishing?' I asked.
>
> "'Today we will just stay home,' someone answered.
>
> "'Aren't you hungry?'
>
> "'Pirahãs aren't eating every day. Pirahãs are hard. Americans eat a lot. Pirahãs eat little.'
>
> "Pirahãs consider hunger a useful tool to toughen themselves. Missing a meal or two, or even going without eating for a day, is taken in stride. I have seen people dance for three days with only brief breaks, not hunting, fishing, or gathering—without any stockpiled food."[3]

Everett later notes that when he brings a few Pirahã into a Brazilian town with restaurants, they gain 20 to 30 pounds in a matter of weeks—their systems quickly succumb to the abundance of rich foods available. However, upon returning to the village, their rolls of belly fat quickly disappear.

Let's all go back to the village.

NOTES

1 The quote is from the chapter "Experiments in Dietetics." The chapter chronicles Gandhi's life when he left India to study law in London. During those years he first experimented with vegetarianism. Prior to the mainstream interest in vegetarianism that began in the 1960s, vegetarianism then was a considered a method for simplifying life and reducing appetites, expectations, and consumption. Mohandas K. Gandhi, *Autobiography: The Story of My Experiments with Truth* (Boston, Mass: Beacon Press, 1993), 56.

2 Jonathan Swift, *Gulliver's Travels,* Part IV, Chapter 2. (1726).

3 Daniel Everett, *Don't Sleep, There Are Snakes: Life and Language in the Amazonian Jungle* (New York: Vintage Departures, 2009), 76.

CHAPTER 15

Return to Nicaragua

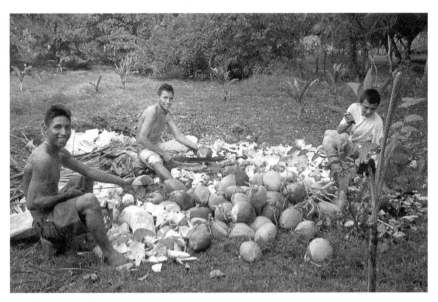

Teenage boys perform the first step in processing coconuts, using machetes to slice away and remove the thick woody husks. *(Padre Ramos)*

Coca-Cola K-Os Coconuts

In 2006 my graduate school awarded me a grant to fund a summer of studying nutrition and health in Nicaragua. For one of my projects, I spent a week with an ecotourism nonprofit venture in Padre Ramos, a coastal village tucked between the Pacific Ocean and a string of estuaries that are part of Nicaragua's national park system. Among our goals was to help the owners of a palm-thatched, open-air restaurant/convenience store make it more attractive to foreign tourists. I worked with the restaurant staff first on food-safety basics like having a place to wash their hands and covering their hair while cooking. Later our group worked on writing a tourist-friendly menu and on preventing the owners' refrigerator-size pig from roaming into the dining area.

I was surprised to find that the store, despite its remote location, sold imported products like instant noodles, mayonnaise, catsup, crackers, chips, candy, and vegetable oils. More surprising was the discovery that the only beverage the restaurant served was Coca-Cola.

I'd noticed that right next door to the restaurant was a small family business that processed coconuts. One afternoon I was seeking alternative refreshment and hopped over the waist-high fence between the properties. I followed the sound of salsa music to the backyard, where I saw three teenage boys. They were singing along to the radio and swaying in a seated dance as they sliced the thick green husks from a large pile of coconuts. To get their attention I waved my hands and shouted out a hearty "Buenos días!"

"Excuse me, how much for a liter of coconut water?" I inquired of the nearest fellow, while shaking my empty water bottle.

"You want what? *Coconut water?*" From his bemused expression I could tell that I might as well have asked him to fill my bottle with sand.

After a few minutes of chatter, and considerable laughter on his part, we struck a deal. He filled my bottle with coconut water and gave me a large bowl full of chopped coconut meat. As I snacked and drank my tropical treat he explained his surprised reaction. No one he knew liked the taste of coconut water, and he couldn't recall the last time he saw someone eating coconut. Because there was no local demand, Padre Ramos sent its coconut harvest to the nearest city (Léon) to be processed and exported.

The most striking part of his story was this revelation: because coconuts are so common in most of the country, they are valued at only a few pennies each. Meanwhile, a bottle of Coke cost 40 cents. In spite of the abundance of this local resource — and the price difference between the drinks — *nobody* in the village drank coconut water. Many villagers (whose income averaged one to two dollars a day) drank Coke at least a few times a week. Teenagers would even fill empty Coke bottles with water so that they could proudly strut through town feigning wealth.

In that case, I'd like the world to buy *me* a Coke. Assuming an average daily salary in the USA of approximately $200, a (rural) Nicaraguan buying a 40-cent Coke is equivalent to an American buying a $40 beverage.

This unsettling discovery led me to survey every Nicaraguan I met about his or her beverage preferences. *In hundreds of interviews I never once encountered a Nicaraguan who favored coconut water.* When not drinking Coke or other imported beverages, they drank sweetened beverages made in Latin America, coffee, heavily sweetened homemade juices, corn-based drinks, or, as a last resort, water. At the restaurant, it took me several days of cajoling to convince my skeptical hosts that if they put coconut water on the menu foreign tourists would happily buy it. Nicas from all over the country were in near universal agreement that coconuts are a primitive, old-fashioned food, often using the word *indio* to describe them. The literal translation is Indian (indigenous), but the word is used to imply poverty, ignorance, and the lowest socioeconomic status—like the English words redneck, yokel, or hayseed.

"Que Indio!" Indio is also used to describe anything of low quality, like a cheap pair of flip-flops that fall apart after a month—or when you do something dumb, like forget an appointment or hit your thumb with a hammer.

At the other end of the popularity spectrum, the overwhelming favorite was Coke. The most common explanations I heard for Coke's appeal were that it was cool, modern, sophisticated; it tasted great; and it made one feel energetic and happy. Coke also served an important function in social gatherings. Several Nicas gave me variations on this party-planning tip:

> "If you want to have a successful party it is important that people see you at the store buying Coke. Don't put the bottles in a bag—you have to carry them in your arms so everyone sees you walking home with them. By the time you are home the word will have spread and all your friends and neighbors will show up, excited about the party."

Persuading people to give up a free, health-sustaining, traditional beverage in favor of spending as much as one-fifth of their daily income on a few pennies worth of caffeinated sugar water is nothing short of modern-day sorcery. What is the recipe for this potent spell? Well-designed and omnipresent advertising: a dash of radio, a splash of billboards, a sprinkling of newspaper, and a steady stream of TV.

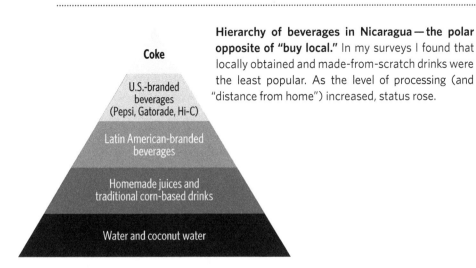

Hierarchy of beverages in Nicaragua — the polar opposite of "buy local." In my surveys I found that locally obtained and made-from-scratch drinks were the least popular. As the level of processing (and "distance from home") increased, status rose.

Coke

U.S.-branded beverages (Pepsi, Gatorade, Hi-C)

Latin American-branded beverages

Homemade juices and traditional corn-based drinks

Water and coconut water

Nutritional Colonialism

"He may be a son of a bitch, but he's our son of a bitch."
PRESIDENT FRANKLIN D. ROOSEVELT, ON ANASTASIO SOMOZA

How did Coca-Cola come to conquer the coconut? While national dietary shifts happen over many generations — even centuries — a watershed year for Nicaragua was 1936. That year Anastasio Somoza García (whom the U.S. had installed as head of the National Guard several years prior) ousted President Adolfo Díaz and founded what was to become a dictatorial dynasty.* Somoza and the small upper class that filled the professional ranks (lawyers, doctors, engineers, administrators, accountants, and military officers) were of European descent and their aspirations aligned with the Western mindset. The priority of the elite was modernization of the country: power plants and electrification, importation of modern goods (tractors, cars, radios, refrigerators), installation of telephone lines, and paving of roads.

To design and implement these aims, Nicaragua's elite collaborated with U.S. leaders in government and business. Their plan to finance the modernization was to generate export products using two resources Nicaragua had in abundance: its land and the labor of indigenous and *mestizo* subsistence farmers. During the 43-year Somoza dictatorship, many farmers were removed from their ancestral lands to make room for the large-scale production of export products (beef, cotton, coffee, tobacco, sugar, bananas, and chocolate) and raw materials (timber, rubber, gold, and other minerals). Cumulatively, these actions modernized parts of the country, created a small middle class, enriched the upper classes, and delivered a substantial profit to U.S. companies. The greatest beneficiary, however, was Anastasio Somoza García. By the 1950s he had become one of the richest men in all of Central America.

While the elite prospered, many of the working class and poor suffered. In their shift from subsistence living to working in an export-oriented economy, most no longer had the time or land to cultivate their traditional diet. The results were severe. Public health assessments estimated that from one-third to well over half the population suffered from malnutrition.[1] This, together with revelations of endemic government corruption and numerous human rights violations, led to the Somozas being viewed by the international community as despots. Additionally, disenfranchised workers were proving to be fertile recruitment material for an increasingly powerful group of land-reform-oriented revolutionaries, the Sandinistas.

* Three different Somozas ruled from 1936-1979.

In a move to reverse malnutrition rates and to quell both domestic unrest and foreign critics, Nicaragua's government cooperated with international aid groups. With the help of USAID, the Institute of Nutrition of Central America and Panama, and the Alliance for Progress (a 1960s-era initiative of President Kennedy), the government promoted the production and consumption of foods that were cheap, calorie dense, and shelf-stable. The most consequential of these were sugar, white rice, and vegetable oil.

Authorities did *not* emphasize fruits and vegetables because they were (and are) more expensive per calorie than other commodities, they spoil quickly, and their low calorie content makes them of little use in preventing calorie malnutrition. While the public health efforts were instrumental in preventing widespread hunger, the solution for one era—weight-promoting, calorie-dense, shelf-stable foods—planted the seed for an epidemic in the next era.

Vegetable oil was a particularly ingenious dietary innovation. In Nicaragua its origin was as a by-product of cotton processing — pressing otherwise worthless cotton seeds for oil.

....

Four Dietary Stages of Central America

1	2	3	4

DIETARY STAGE	TIMELINE	KEY FOODS
1 Hunter-Gatherer	From 20,000 BCE	game, seafood, wild-gathered plants *(grains, legumes, seeds, tubers)*
2 Whole-Foods Agrarian	From 7,000 BCE–present	beans, corn, vegetables
3 Processed Agrarian	Mid-20th century–present	white rice, vegetable oil, sugar
4 Modern Processed	URBAN: 1990s–present RURAL: 2000s–present	processed food and drink, and factory-farmed animal products

When humans arrived in the Americas they were hunter-gatherers. Two factors—the hunting of big game into scarcity (and often extinction) and rising population density—fueled the transition to the more productive (more calories per acre) agrarian diet.

The original whole-foods version of the agrarian diet dominated until the mid-20th century, when post-WWII advances in farming, food processing, and transportation made possible widespread access to vegetable oil, sugar, and white rice. Over time, these three alone replaced more than half of the calories in the traditional agrarian diet.

In the early 1990s Nicaragua's first post-civil-war president, Violeta Chamorro, signed economic and trade agreements intended to bring the country back into the global economy. Those agreements, expanded by later administrations, sparked the import of modern processed foods into urban areas and, in the last decade, rural areas as well.

....

Nicaragua's Dietary Transition

A Glimpse Back to the Whole-Foods Agrarian Diet

It might surprise you that Nicaragua, the second-poorest country in Latin America, could have an obesity epidemic in 2017. How rapidly things change! When I first visited the country in 2002 it had just emerged from a century in which the primary public health concern had been the prevention of hunger and calorie malnutrition.

I made that first trip with a volunteer group working on a solar energy project in Las Pintadas, a high mountain village within walking distance of the Honduran border.[2] Remote even by Nicaraguan standards, it was reachable only after hours of travel by off-road vehicle, followed by a walk or horse ride up the mountain. Unlike Padre Ramos, the village had no running water and no electricity. Villagers were exposed to external media only when the mayor occasionally hooked up an old 12-volt black-and-white TV to a borrowed car battery.

Our group included an obese young man, Elliot. While a group of foreigners always attracts attention, the villagers couldn't take their eyes off Elliot. Children wanted to touch his stomach and teenagers gossiped about him as if he were a celebrity. "He must be a politician." "I heard he owns two houses." The stir Elliot caused wasn't surprising; he was surely the first obese person most of the villagers had ever seen. In 2002 obesity was beginning to be a factor in Nicaraguan cities, but was still exceptionally rare in the most rural parts of the country.

The people of Las Pintadas were slim and fit. They woke up before the sun rose, and when it set they lit a pinkie-sized candle, told a few stories, and were in bed moments after the last light flickered away. In between they reaped, sowed, and cared for their animals. In their free time they played soccer and baseball, sang, danced, and prayed. There were no roads, so they walked everywhere and rode horses where it was possible. A few times a year they took some of their harvest to a neighboring village to trade it for the few necessities of life they could not provide for themselves, primarily clothing, tools, and medicine.

Their diet was barely affected by the 20th century—even aid programs rarely came as far as their village. More than half of their calories came from corn and beans; vegetables and fruit also made a significant contribution. With the exception of the eggs they ate almost daily (everyone raised chickens), animal foods were a small, infrequent part of their diet. When a chicken got too old to lay eggs, it was eaten. For villagers handy with a slingshot, rabbit or iguana occasionally provided a meaty side dish.

Furthermore, the nearest store was at least an hour's ride on horseback, so sugar, oil, rice, and flour made only occasional appearances in their diet. Not just inconvenient to obtain, these foods were also too expensive to be daily staples. And, finally, junk food was a rare novelty, something brought into the village a few times a year.

Processed Agrarian and Modern Processed Diets

I spent 2014, via a Fulbright Scholar grant, as a visiting professor with the Universidad Nacional Autónoma de Nicaragua. I was awarded the grant to develop a nutrition curriculum and to teach courses with an emphasis on obesity and chronic disease. At that time obesity had reached epidemic levels in Nicaragua, with well over half the adult population either overweight or obese.[3]

> Nicaragua's experience with obesity is typical not only of Latin America, but of most of the developing world. From Kenya to India to Papua New Guinea, obesity rates have skyrocketed in the past few decades.

All of my fellow nutrition professors were Nicaraguan. They were a talented, well-educated group, but having grown up in the Nicaragua of the 1980s and '90s, they had little experience with obesity and chronic disease. They had spent their careers developing and applying medical nutrition therapies for conditions that result from calorie and nutrient deficiencies: anemia, low-birth-weight infants, underweight pregnancies, vitamin A deficiency, and protein deficiency. I taught classes on weight management to these professors as well as to students and nutrition professionals. I explained the USA's struggle with weight, the numerous root causes, and the benefits and drawbacks to various weight loss strategies. Together we brainstormed solutions for Nicaragua. I also taught cooking classes and physical activity classes, and worked with local non-profit and government groups on type 2 diabetes.

Outside my classrooms, I became the student. I observed and compared diets in Managua and each of the other villages and cities I visited, scribbling down notes and taking photos. This was my sixth extended stay in Nicaragua since 2002 (intervening trips were in 2006, 2008, 2010, and 2012) and the pattern was becoming as predictable as the sunrise: every year the Nicaraguan diet became more Westernized. Not coincidentally, this period of expanding girth was matched by a gradually improving economy. It seemed that every additional dollar in income added an inch to the nation's collective waistline. By 2014 Nicaraguan diets were bursting with white rice, sugar, soda, bread, pastries, chips, and candy—and more oil, meat, and cheese than ever before.

Three Nicaraguan Diets at a Glance

As the percentage of processed food increases, calorie density and overall calorie intake rise.

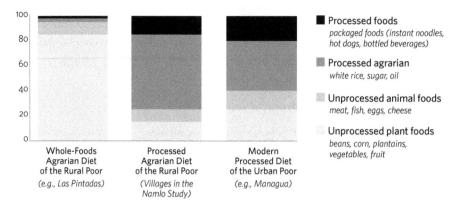

■ **Processed foods**
packaged foods (instant noodles, hot dogs, bottled beverages)

■ **Processed agrarian**
white rice, sugar, oil

■ **Unprocessed animal foods**
meat, fish, eggs, cheese

Unprocessed plant foods
beans, corn, plantains, vegetables, fruit

Whole-Foods Agrarian Diet of the Rural Poor	Processed Agrarian Diet of the Rural Poor	Modern Processed Diet of the Urban Poor
(e.g., Las Pintadas)	*(Villages in the Namlo Study)*	*(e.g., Managua)*

While the *progression* of the urban diet didn't surprise me, I hadn't spent enough time in the far-flung reaches of the country to know how *pervasive* the issue was. At the end of my tenure at UNAN I got the opportunity to fill that gap via a joint venture between the university and Namlo, a nonprofit based in Denver, Colorado.

Namlo hired me to design a survey to assess the diets, health, and socioeconomic status of Nicaraguans in five poor, isolated communities. In addition to collecting dietary, anthropometric, and economic data, I included 20 questions to assess Nicas' general knowledge about nutrition. Then, with the help of four of my UNAN nutrition students I surveyed 50 families (200 people in total).

Many Nicas expressed the belief that all food is healthy. Few understood that some foods have deleterious consequences, and often assumed that processed foods were superior to local foods. For instance, they rated cornflakes and milk as healthier than beans and tortillas, and in general didn't rate vegetables as any better or worse than processed foods like chips. They also didn't understand that diet and lifestyle are connected to disease. This is consistent with other research on Latin America, where a fatalistic view of health dominates. When asked about what determines whether one is healthy or not, the most common response is *"qué Dios quiere"* (what God wants). One connection participants occasionally made was between modern food and cavities. People over 70 years old regularly commented that theirs was the first generation to have cavities, which have become more common with every subsequent generation.

In the results of the survey it was possible to see the details of the transition from the traditional diet (beans, corn, vegetables). My team found that about 30 percent of the calories in participants' diets came from white rice, 15 percent from sugar, 15 percent from vegetable oil, and at least 15 percent from packaged processed foods and beverages (instant noodles, soda, candy etc.). The convenience store filled with processed foods was once an urban species; it was now ubiquitous, popping up in even the most remote villages.

Snapshots from the Road

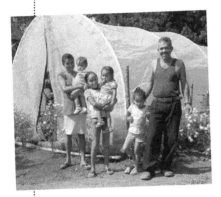

Las Palmas

Namlo works with communities to improve their diets and provide a sustainable income. One program teaches organic gardening using inexpensive shade cloth greenhouses. This has been more successful than originally anticipated. In 2016, 76 families produced $39,500 (USD) worth of organic produce. The families eat a portion of the harvest (boosting their nutrition intake), but most is sold through an organic marketplace that Namlo developed.

Barrio Nuevo

Rural Nicaraguan culture isn't number-oriented, so very few of my interview subjects knew their height or weight. A few people even had to check their government ID cards to remind them of their age.

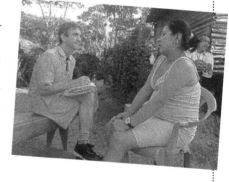

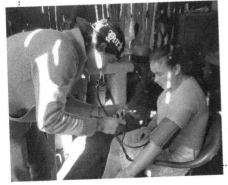

El Quebracho.

Diego Gabriel Castro Navarro, one of my nutrition students, takes the blood pressure of one our research subjects.

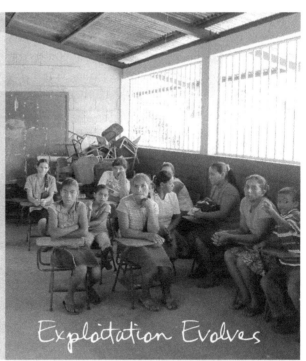

Nicaragua's poverty is most apparent in its education system, as the average Nicaraguan's education is equivalent to the sixth-grade level in North America. Few Nicas have the scientific literacy to understand the connection between diet and health. As Nicaraguan nutritionists often lamented to me, **Nicas learn about food through marketing, not in school.** One of the truisms of public health is that in populations with access to a modern diet, education level is the most accurate predictor of health outcomes — i.e., the less education one has, the greater one's risk of disease.

Exploitation Evolves

Capitalism Gone Feral

The 1990s marked a tipping point in tobacco use in the United States. As awareness of the negative effects of smoking rose, public opinion pushed the federal government to stiffly regulate and even successfully sue the tobacco industry. The industry responded by exploring markets in the developing world, where weaker governments would not put up roadblocks and where uneducated people could be convinced, via marketing, that cigarettes were modern, exciting status symbols.

In recent years, as Americans are starting to question and even regulate processed foods, the food industry is following the same international strategy set by tobacco.

FOUR STAGES OF CONQUEST

	1

At one time the conquistadors, colonial powers, and dictators of Latin America's past used the threat of violence to extract value from the poor. Now people exchange their minimal resources (and health) for both seductive processed foods and the expensive solutions to treat the diseases they bring about.

Select a minimally educated population ideally led by a weak, naive, or complicit government

Unhealthy for the Body, Unhealthy for the Country

In rural areas a common sight is a farmer ambling up to a convenience store with a few chickens and a basket of produce to exchange for soda, vegetable oil, and candy. Meanwhile, northern-bound ships leave Nicaraguan ports packed with valuable raw agriculture products: coffee, beef, shrimp, lobster, timber, chocolate, tobacco, and a variety of fruits and vegetables. These ships return with calorie-dense processed foods. These **lopsided exchanges** are not just a Nicaraguan phenomenon, but are symbolic of the relationship between developing countries and the developed world.

Perhaps the most striking example of edible exploitation is the infant formula scandal of the 20th century. In the 1960s, Nestlé and Bristol-Myers began to aggressively market infant formula in Latin America and Africa, promoting it as modern, sophisticated, and nutritionally superior to breastfeeding. Whatever the motivation for these campaigns, the result was a staggering increase in infant mortality. Mothers couldn't always afford sufficient formula, and once a mother stops breastfeeding it is almost impossible to begin again. Exacerbating the issue was the inconsistent availability of potable water needed to make the formula; the use of poor-quality water in the mix caused widespread diarrhea and infant death. A broad coalition of international aid groups, humanitarian organizations, and world governments eventually pressured the infant formula industry to adopt strict marketing restrictions. The restrictions were combined with highly effective public health campaigns promoting breastfeeding, which once again became the preferred way to feed infants.

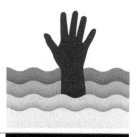

2	3	4
Market rich food or other addictive substances as status symbols (cigarettes and alcohol are also examples)	When the health of the people weakens, **market processed food and supplements as panaceas** (energy drinks, vitamin pills, fortified cereals, protein powder, superfoods)	When disease arrives **sell the "solution"**: pharmaceutical drugs, surgery, and other medical interventions.

In total, nearly two thirds of our survey participants' calories came from white rice, sugar, and oil. The average family of five in our survey population bought, at minimum, one liter of vegetable oil, five pounds of sugar, and 10 pounds of rice per week. None of these foods had been consumed in significant quantity prior to the 20th century. These "new" foods are calorie dense, which ensured that these rural populations had low incidences of calorie malnutrition—no one in our survey group was starving. We saw only a handful of people who were a little underweight; meanwhile, overweight and obesity were almost as high as in Nicaragua's cities. Our analysis showed, however, that this calorie-dense diet was deficient in vitamins A, B6, B12, and E and almost all minerals. Although most nutrient deficiencies don't have visible

Rice, sugar, and oil took decades to become staples in Nicaragua. The older people I interviewed about their childhood diets reported that neither they nor their peers consumed rice or vegetable oil, and that sugar and other sweets were rarities.

symptoms, we noted a high frequency of a few common signs, including cracks at the corners of the mouth, ridged nails, coarse, brittle hair, and pale skin. We also noted growth stunting in some children—not from a lack of calories but from vitamin and mineral deficiencies.

Naïve to Consequence: We Can't Believe It Til We See It

In Western societies a critical mass of people has struggled with the debilitating complications of excess weight: disease, medication, surgery, and debt. This shared experience has given us a visceral understanding of the impacts of diet and lifestyle.

The developing world is rapidly catching up, but people do not yet have the same history of struggle with weight. Very few understand that the quality of one's diet can lead either to good health and relative ease in mid- to later life or to pain, discomfort, and disease. Until recently, extra weight was still considered a sign of status. Although that perception is changing, a bulging belly is still viewed as relatively benign when compared to the crippling diseases of scarcity that marked the recent past.

Universal Root Causes

History repeats itself, but with an ironic twist. While Nicaragua has far fewer problems with calorie scarcity then it did in the 20th century, the diseases brought about by excess calories (most notably diabetes and cardiovascular disease) could prove even harder to resolve. If the trends of the last few decades continue, worker productivity will drop, medical expenses will bankrupt the country, and the resulting economic turmoil could, once again, provoke civil unrest.

While the myriad causes of the obesity epidemic are too numerous to cover, two main factors are common all over the globe: a change in food culture and less physical activity.[4]

Nicaraguans are in the midst of a rapid transition from a whole-foods agrarian diet to processed agrarian and modern processed diets. Along with the diets, they are adopting a Western perspective on food: as entertainment, as a mood-altering substance, and as a means to obtain and express social status.

Fewer and fewer Nicaraguans are following a traditional life, with many hours of walking and physically demanding agricultural work. Increasingly they work in factories, the service/tourist industry, call centers, and warehouses. Additionally, entertainment options, once largely physical in nature (dancing and sports), are now more sedentary (TV, the internet, video games).

The Solution

In 1979 Nicaragua broke free of 43 years of the Somoza family dictatorship. The repressive Somoza years were followed by a U.S.-backed civil war in the 1980s that brought widespread bloodshed and a devastating economic depression. In the early 1990s the country began and has sustained a period of relative stability, peace, and economic growth. The working class finally has a few coins to jingle together and no fear of imminent disaster, which means people are in the mood for a feast. In the current environment a dietitian feels much like a priest who stumbles upon a wild orgy, and, overwhelmed, exclaims "The path you take leads to ruin! Turn down that racket and put on your clothes! You are all going to get venereal disease and lose your soul!"

Instead of begging people to drop the "infant formula" that is modern foods, a more effective tactic would be empowering Nicaraguans through education; promoting the "breast milk" that is a local, unprocessed diet. Specifically, education should address the questions that Nicaragua and much of the developing world faces, including:

Biology...	What are the nutritional needs of the people?
	How do changing diets and lifestyles affect Nicaraguans?
Economics...	What are the consequences of exporting raw agricultural goods and importing processed foods?
	Are Nicaraguans, on a local and a national level, in danger of ceding their food sovereignty and economic independence?
Psychology...	How are marketers manipulating the public?
	How does social pressure play a role in food choices?
	What are the benefits and drawbacks to modern and traditional perspectives on diet?
Environment...	How does changing dietary patterns and an export-focused economy impact agricultural patterns and the long-term productivity of the land?
Government...	Is the obligation of government to protect the uneducated?
	Can food marketing be regulated?
	What is the most effective way to deliver nutrition education to the public?

Always Befriend Your Neighbor

In March 2015 I traveled to the last town in my nutrition survey. My destination, Los Pinares, was in the high mountains of Madriz state, which makes up the border region between Nicaragua and Honduras. The steep dirt road twisted and turned for hours, and our jampacked 1970s school bus sputtered, groaned, and rattled every inch of the way. As my stomach churned, I chuckled at the irony that, in my twenties, I used to relish demanding journeys to mountaintops; then I felt sure that every peak would reward my effort with some deeper understanding of the universe.

To take my mind off my nausea, I chatted with the fellow seated next to me. Vicente, a former Sandinista revolutionary in his seventies, was still in fine shape. He told me about his current work teaching people living in the mountains how to use greenhouses to grow organic vegetables, thoughtfully explaining the project's health and ecological benefits. As we reached the summit and began to unload, he said, with a knowing smile, "Amigo, the United States could also benefit from small-scale organic gardening."

I began this book with a story about a different neighbor's advice. In the 1980s, in Washington, D.C., my parents' wealthy neighbor in an affluent section of the city had advised another former revolutionary soldier, my father, to stop growing vegetables in our front yard. She was concerned that our chaotic garden might prevent us from fitting into our refined surroundings. That story of neighborly conflict eventually led to friendship. But will the story of our relationship with our global neighbors end in friendship? Or will the transnational food companies and the politicians they influence continue to ignore the well-being of the populace in developing nations next door?

Like our well-heeled D.C. neighbor, those of us with the power to change what is on the table should look over the fence and befriend our neighbors. In learning about their history and traditions we might find a basket of vegetables fresh from the garden, and along with it, a new perspective for us all.

As for me, I will listen to Vicente.

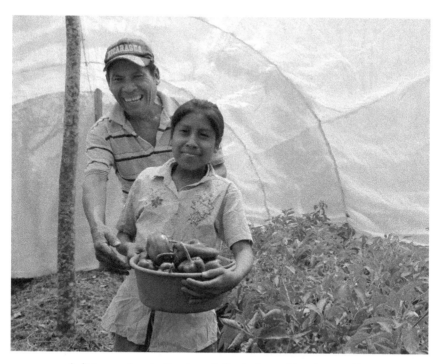

A dietary and agricultural revolution in the making: Jose and his daughter Elena in their mountaintop greenhouse in Los Pinares

NOTES

1 Detailed information on Nicaraguan public health history is not abundant, but the sources listed here offer two perspectives. Christiane Berth offers an excellent, broad overview in her article "Food Policy and Consumption in Nicaragua 1965-1995" in the *Dialogues Electronic Journal of History* 15(1), February-August 2014. You'll find a detailed snapshot of healthcare in the mid-1970s in USAID's report *USAID Nutrition Assessment Sector for Nicaragua* (USAID: Managua, Nicaragua, May 14, 1976).

2 I talked about Las Pintadas in the "Conversations in Nicaragua" feature in Chapter 2 (page 23). I also chronicled my trip in the October/November 2003 issue of *Home Power Magazine*.

3 Timothy Luax et al., "Prevalence of obesity, tobacco use, and alcohol consumption by socio-economic status among six communities in Nicaragua." *Pan American Journal of Public Health* 32 (2012), 217–255.

4 Tucker Bermudez and Katherine Tucker, "Trends in dietary patterns of Latin American populations" *Reports in Public Health*, 2003; 19 Suppl 1: S87-99. Epub 2003 July 21; Lisa Pawloski et al., "The Nutrition Transition: Evidence from Nicaragua, Costa Rica, and Chile," *Global Studies Review* Vol. 6, No. 2, Summer 2010.

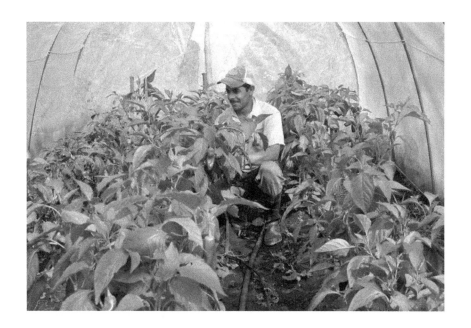

Appendix

The Dieter's Essentials | Recipes and Cooking Tips

The Dieter's Essentials

CONVENIENT LOW-CALORIE FOODS

CATEGORY	EXAMPLES	NOTES
Vegetables		
Raw	jicama, peppers, carrots, celery, tomatoes, Jerusalem artichoke, sugar snap peas	These are ideal for snacks on their own, or paired with a low-calorie dip (see hummus and black bean dip recipes, page 194).
Dried or dehydrated	all kinds; purchase premade or DIY in the oven (you'll find methods online)	Use these to add flavor and chewy texture. They're so easy to add to soups and stews and taste great.
Easy-to-cook starchy	pumpkin, squash, sweet potatoes, corn, potatoes	When you need a filling starch these require minimal effort.
Sea	dulse, wakame, kelp, kombu, sea lettuce, nori	These add a complex umami flavor to all kinds of meals. Use them to make broth; add to beans and salads.
Canned soups	miso, lentil, and bean	Handy for the occasional quick meal or meal addition. (Their high salt content means that they shouldn't be daily staples.)
Fruit	fresh, frozen, and canned	Fresh fruit is your best choice, but it's great to have options. Keep around for a stand-alone snack or mix with yogurt for something more filling.
Mushrooms	chanterelle, portobello, oyster, straw, shiitake	Mushrooms add a unique meaty flavor. Try them roasted or in soup.

CONDIMENTS

Use low-calorie condiments to add flavor to your Sober Plate meals. Good examples are puréed tomatoes, salsa, nutritional yeast, hot sauce, soy sauce, mustard, vinegar; and don't forget homemade or store-bought low-calorie sauces, marinades, and dressings.

There are condiment suggestions on page 42 and marinade recipes on page 205.

CITRUS

The strong acidic flavor of citrus highlights the flavors of many dishes. Citrus can be used as both a marinade and a topping. Try a squeeze of lime, lemon, or orange on meat, fish, beans, vegetables, and almost every kind of fruit. (Lemon juice on watermelon is my favorite.)

KITCHENWARE

Plate size is a strong influence on the portions we serve ourselves. Big plates, bowls, and utensils are a visual cue to eat more; small ones, a cue to eat less. For home use, choose smaller plates (nine inches or less), as well as smaller bowls, glasses, and cutlery.

Use the trick employed by all-you-can-eat restaurants — they supply small plates to prompt their patrons to eat less.

NONSTICK COOKWARE

There is a wide variety of nonstick cookware available, made from minerals and ceramics that are durable and entirely nontoxic. For the dieter, the ability to sauté and heat food with little or no fat makes these tools essential. (Also, knowing that clean-up will take only minutes adds the extra incentive to do your own healthy cooking.)

> TIP: *Hand wash your nonstick cookware rather than putting it in the dishwasher. It only takes a minute, and will ensure a longer life for both the nonstick surface and the cookware.*

RICE COOKER

This time-saving device costs about 20 or 30 dollars. You can even find decent used models at thrift shops for just a few dollars. Look for models with a non-aluminum interior — ceramic or stainless steel is best. If you like cooking your vegetables and grains together, look for a model with a built-in second level.

Then, throw in your favorite grains, some low-sodium bouillon (or, better yet, a few herbs), and you can cook with minimal effort.

> TIP: *Keep in mind that grains and vegetables have differing cooking times. For instance, when you make a long-cooking grain like brown rice (which needs about 30 minutes) wait until the last five minutes of cooking time to add a quick-cooking veggie like asparagus.*

CROCK-POT/SLOW COOKER

These are the lazy cook's best friend — you can make slimming meals with ease. Use the same proportion of ingredients in the slow cooker that you would when making any other Sober Plate meal: half nonstarchy veggies, one-quarter starch, and one-quarter protein.

> TIP: *Slow cooking is ideal for lean cuts of meat — the low, slow heat ensures that it will stay tender and juicy.*

STEAMER

Steaming — whether you use a steamer basket in a pot on the stovetop or an electric steamer — is one of the easiest ways to prepare vegetables. Steaming retains the original color, taste, and volume of vegetables.

> TIP: *Add spices to the water in your steamer to both enhance flavor and make your kitchen smell great. There are many good-quality electric steamers on the market for under 40 dollars.*

ELECTRIC OR GEORGE FOREMAN GRILL

These grills are fun and easy to use. There is no need to add oil to the grill surface and everything cooks in a few minutes.

> TIP: *Marinate protein and vegetables for at least 20 minutes before cooking. The marinade will provide flavor and help prevent the food from sticking.*

MICROWAVE

Though microwaves alter the taste and texture of many foods, particularly those that contain a low percentage of water (bread, bagels), many dieters love their convenience for reheating leftovers.

HOT-AIR POPCORN POPPER

With a hot-air popper you control the calories and the fat and salt content, by starting with popcorn kernels and hot air.

TIP: *For a sweet, low-calorie snack, top fresh, hot popcorn with some cinnamon mixed with a little stevia powder or xylitol. For a savory taste, mist with a light coating of olive oil and sprinkle with a mix of seasonings or dried herbs (like the Mrs. Dash mixtures).*

FOOD PROCESSOR

Chopping, grating, and slicing vegetables by hand can get tedious. Food processors get the job done quickly and easily, and their interchangeable blades allow for a variety of different shapes and textures. There are many processors and mini-choppers available for less than 50 dollars.

ADVANCE PREP AND STORAGE, THE BUSY DIETER'S BEST FRIEND

Keeping an array of storage containers on hand makes it convenient to prepare food in quantity when you have time—on the weekend, for instance. This allows you to have healthy meals (either to very quickly assemble and cook or to easily reheat) during your busy workweek. I prefer glass or Pyrex containers because they last forever and take heat well, but plastic containers also work.

On Sunday evenings I cook a few meals for the week. Sometimes I make brown rice and beans; other times I only make the protein. I always shred several cups of vegetables in my food processor. Once I'm done I portion the food into containers. I refrigerate some to eat during the week, and freeze some for later.

NOTES

Pay attention to temperatures:

- Refrigerate raw vegetables until you're ready to use them.
- Cool hot foods to room temperature before you freeze them.

Store:

- Mind the gap: Don't leave too much space—air in the container can cause freezer burn. For foods with significant water content, leave about ¾ inches between the food and the lid (the water will expand when it freezes). For drier items, squeeze out as much air as you can before you seal the container.
- Use the smallest container that makes sense. The faster food freezes, the fresher it will taste when you heat it up again.

RECIPES and COOKING TIPS

I developed these recipes while teaching culinary classes at Wellspring Weight Loss Camps and at Shane Diet & Fitness Resorts. I also used many of these same recipes in Nicaragua when I taught cooking classes to my nutrition students.

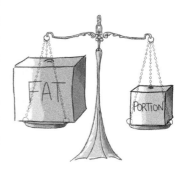

All of these recipes are low in fat and offer a con-siderable portion size for the modest number of calories. You always have the option of increasing the fat and reducing the portion size.

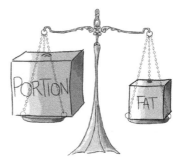

Healthy Snacks

> Beans are an excellent vegetarian protein choice for weight loss.

BLACK BEAN DIP/SPREAD

This dip goes well with tortilla chips (baked, of course!) and fresh veggies. It is a good sandwich spread, too.

2 cans (15-ounce) black beans, rinsed and drained

¼ medium red onion

3 Roma tomatoes

2 garlic cloves

3 tablespoons chopped fresh cilantro

1 tablespoon lime juice

½ tablespoon balsamic vinegar

1 teaspoon cumin

½ teaspoon salt

¼ teaspoon cayenne pepper

Place all ingredients in a food processor fitted with a metal blade. Process until it's the consistency you like—a little chunky or puréed until smooth. Add sea salt to taste, garnish with extra cilantro. Do not eat cold; this dip tastes best at room temperature.

HEALTHY HOMEMADE HUMMUS

While you can find low- and nonfat hummus at the grocery store (Cedar's, Skinny Girl, and Engine 2 are worth a try) this homemade recipe is tastier and far less expensive. It will stay fresh for at least one week in the refrigerator.

1 red bell pepper, chopped

1 small eggplant, cut into 1-inch cubes

3 cloves garlic, peeled

1 teaspoon olive oil

2 cups chickpeas

⅓ cup broth (vegetarian or chicken)

2 teaspoons ground cumin

2 teaspoons soy sauce
(Bragg Liquid Aminos is even better)

1 lemon, juiced

Salt and pepper

Preheat the oven to 425°F. Put the pepper, eggplant, and garlic on a nonstick or parchment paper-lined sheet pan, and give them tiny spritz of vegetable oil. Roast until soft and cooked through, about 10-15 minutes. Put the roasted vegetables, chickpeas, broth, garlic, cumin, and soy sauce into the work bowl of a food processor. Add the lemon juice. Process until the mixture becomes a thick paste. Season to taste with salt and pepper.

TIP: *Use hummus as a dip for vegetables—or as the protein in a sandwich: add sliced tomatoes, lettuce, and red onion for a great combination.*

Both recipes
Serving size: 2 tablespoons. Makes 30 servings.
Per serving: 30 calories; <0.5 grams fat

Salads, Slaws, Sides

THE RESISTANT STARCH SALAD

There are many variations on this salad — experiment with different combinations from the lists in the table below. Pick one or two starches, one or two proteins, and three or four vegetables.

	Vegetables	Starches	Protein		
Cooking options	Steam until slightly soft	Bake, boil, steam, or roast		Vegetables (raw)	Dressing
	green beans, zucchini, squash, nopales	corn, potatoes, rice, pasta, bulgur, barley	beans (*chickpeas are classic but any kind work*), tuna, shellfish, lentils, baked tofu	jicama, carrots, bell peppers, tomatoes, onions, garlic	lime juice (*or any citrus*), cilantro, basil, vinegar (*try a flavor, like fig*), mustard

Use the Sober Plate proportions as a guide: one-quarter protein (3-4 ounces), one-quarter starch (½ to ¾ cup), one-half vegetables (1 cup or more).

Cook and cool your ingredients, then toss together. Top off with a low- or nonfat dressing (use one with less than three grams of fat per two-tablespoon serving).

Serving size: 2-3 cups.
Per serving: 300-400 calories; 2-5 grams fat
Fat and calories will vary with ingredient choices

POWER SALAD

I often made this salad when I lived in Nicaragua, and it was a favorite of Jenny, my illustrator. Jenny would come over in the morning and work, then we would go for a jog or play a little soccer with neighborhood kids. When we returned to my house, still sweating under the tropical sun, this was a filling meal that was ideal when we didn't feel like eating hot food.

4 cups sprouted beans	1 cup chopped cilantro	Salt and pepper
4 cups diced carrots	2 oranges	
4 cups corn	1-2 limes	

Lightly steam beans until they are soft enough to easily chew (if they are still crunchy they can cause gas). Steam or boil carrots and corn until just tender. Put beans, carrots, and corn in a colander and rinse with cold water. Shake the colander to remove the excess water and then put everything in a large serving bowl. Halve the oranges and limes, remove seeds, and squeeze their juice into the bowl. Add cilantro. Mix together all ingredients; add salt and pepper to taste.

Serving size: 3 cups. Makes 4 servings.
Per serving: 409 calories; 2 grams fat

TWO CARROT SALADS

These carrot salads, sweet and savory, are an ideal staple food for weight loss. Kids in particular love the citrus-fruit flavor of the sweet carrot salad.

SWEET ORANGE-CARROT SALAD

6 medium carrots (about 1 pound)

½ cup orange juice concentrate

¼ cup raisins

1 teaspoon ground ginger

Salt to taste

Mix raisins with the concentrate in a small bowl, and let sit for a few minutes to allow the raisins to absorb the orange flavor and become plump. Wash and cut off the tops of the carrots. Feed carrots into a food processor on the grate setting (you can also use a box grater). Mix shredded carrots with the ginger and the juice-raisin mixture, then add salt to taste.

> TIP: *Experiment with other fruit-juice concentrates.*

Serving size: ½ cup. Makes 14 servings.
Per serving: 73 calories; 0 grams fat

SAVORY CARROT SALAD

6 medium carrots

¼ cup chives

¼ cup green onions

Dressing

2 tablespoons balsamic or rice wine vinegar

2 tablespoons chicken broth

1 teaspoon olive oil

1-2 teaspoons mustard

1 tablespoon lemon juice

Salt and pepper to taste

Wash and cut off the tops of the carrots. Feed carrots into a food processor on the grate setting (you can also use a box grater). Dice the onions and cut up the chives (scissors work best); mix in with the carrots. Blend the dressing ingredients in a blender or food processor, then add to the carrot salad.

Serving size: ½ cup. Makes 14 servings.
Per serving: 33 calories; 0.75 grams fat

VEGGIE SLAW

This slaw is a breeze to make in a food processor, but you can use a box grater instead — it'll just take a little longer.

1 medium cabbage

4 medium carrots

1 medium beet

1 small onion

Dressing

¼ cup mustard

2 tablespoons vinegar

2 teaspoons celery seeds

½ teaspoon salt

½ teaspoon pepper

2 tablespoons citrus juice (lime, lemon, orange)

Before beginning, cut the cabbage, onion, and beet into smaller chunks to fit into the feed tube. Cut the carrots lengthwise in half and place in the feed tube in a fairly tight configuration. Feed all ingredients into a food processor fitted with the grating blade. You want to create little "noodles." Process in batches and mix together in a large bowl. In a smaller bowl, whisk together the mustard, vinegar, celery seeds, citrus, salt, and pepper. Pour enough of the dressing over the grated vegetables to moisten them. Serve cold or at room temperature.

> **TIP:** *This is another highly flexible recipe. Try different kinds of cabbage and onions, and vary your veggies: kale, jicama, Jerusalem artichoke, and spring onions are great options. Raisins also make a good addition.*

Serving size: 1 cup. Makes 6 servings.
Per serving: 40 calories; 0 grams fat

MEATY CABBAGE

1 head green cabbage, cored and shredded

1 tablespoon lard or chicken fat, or a thumb-size piece of fatty meat (vegetarians can use vegetable oil)

2 cloves garlic, diced

1 tablespoon caraway seeds

salt, pepper to taste

Heat the fat in a large skillet over medium heat. Once it is hot add the cabbage, garlic, salt, and pepper. Cover with a lid and reduce the heat to medium-low. Cook for about 10 minutes, then sprinkle in the caraway seeds. Cook until fragrant (about 2 minutes).

> **TIP:** *It's important to add the salt early to draw the water out of the cabbage — this assists the cooking process. This dish works well with a touch of plain yogurt.*

Serving size: 1 cup. Makes 4 servings.
Per serving: 60 calories; 4 grams fat

MEATY BAKED FRENCH FRIES/WEDGES

4 large baking potatoes, cut french-fry style or in wedges

1 tablespoon lard, chicken fat, or vegetable oil

1 teaspoon paprika

1 teaspoon garlic powder

1 teaspoon chili powder

½ teaspoon onion powder

Preheat oven to 450°F. Place fat and spices in a large mixing bowl and mix to combine. (If using lard or chicken fat, melt it before mixing in the spices.) Add the potatoes to the bowl and stir to coat with the fat-spice mixture. Using a rubber spatula, turn out the potatoes onto a nonstick or parchment-lined baking sheet; separate and distribute so that the potatoes are in one layer. Bake for about 10 minutes, then flip/stir the fries; continue baking another 10-15 minutes until golden brown.

Serving size: 1 cup. Makes 4 servings.
Per serving: 150 calories; 4 grams fat

Soups

These easy, tasty, nutrient-dense soups use two different low-fat cooking techniques. In the first recipe the ingredients are sautéed before blending, and in the second they are roasted. Both soups can be seasoned with nutritional yeast, a protein that tastes like Parmesan cheese, but is very low in fat and rich in B vitamins, magnesium, and zinc.

30-MINUTE BLACK BEAN SOUP

1 teaspoon oil

2 green bell peppers, stems and seeds removed, diced

1 large onion, diced

2 cloves garlic, minced

¼ jalapeño pepper, stems and seeds removed, minced

½ chipotle pepper, finely minced

1 teaspoon ground cumin

½ teaspoon dried chili flakes

1 quart chicken broth

1 15-ounce can black beans *(not drained)* or 2 cu ps cooked black beans, cooking liquid reserved

2 bay leaves

Low- and no-calorie seasonings:

Cilantro, lime, salt, diced red onion, nutritional yeast *(30 calories per tablespoon)*; plain yogurt; salsa

Heat the oil in a large, nonstick frying pan. When hot, add the green peppers and onions and cook, stirring frequently, until softened but not browned, about 3 minutes. Add the garlic, jalapeño and chipotle, cumin, and dried chili flakes. Cook on medium-high heat, stirring constantly, until fragrant (about 1 minute). Add the chicken broth, the beans and their liquid, and bay leaves. Increase the heat to high and bring to a boil, then reduce to a slow simmer, cover, and cook for 15 minutes.

Discard the bay leaves. Blend, using a blender or food processor, to desired consistency. (Don't blend more than about two cups at a time; it can get messy if you overload the machine.)

Ladle soup into serving bowls and serve immediately. Season at table with any of the seasoning options listed above.

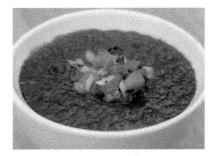

Serving size: 1 cup. Makes 6 servings.
Per serving: 95 calories; <1 gram fat

SQUASH SOUP

4 cups winter squash (butternut, acorn, or delicata), peeled and cut into 1-inch chunks (*about 2 squashes*)

1 apple, peeled, cored, and cut into 1-inch chunks

1 yellow onion, chopped

2-3 cloves garlic, sliced

2 teaspoons ground ginger

3 cups chicken broth

2 tablespoons nutritional yeast

¼ cup chopped fresh parsley

Preheat oven to 400°F. Line a rimmed baking sheet or shallow roasting pan with parchment paper. In a large bowl, toss squash, apples, onion, garlic, and ginger until mixed well. Spread mixture on baking sheets in a single layer and place in oven. Roast until tender and beginning to brown, about 30-45 minutes. (Start checking at 20 minutes to make sure your garlic and apples don't get too crispy.) Remove from oven and purée squash mixture with broth and nutritional yeast in a blender or food processor to desired consistency. Serve garnished with parsley.

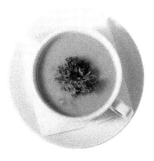

Serving size: 1 cup. Makes 6 servings.
Per serving: 101 calories; 0 grams fat

Main and Small Dishes

SHRIMP CEVICHE

Most ceviche recipes present a problem for dieters because they have too much protein (from the shellfish), not enough vegetables, and often contain high-fat ingredients like avocado or oil. This recipe is well balanced, with enough protein, plenty of vegetables, and almost no fat. It is filling while keeping a low calorie count.

½ pound medium-small shrimp, peeled, deveined, and cut into 1-inch pieces

¾–1 cup lemon or lime juice (*enough to cover the shrimp*)

½ cup red onion, finely chopped

1 cucumber, diced into ½-inch pieces

½ cup jicama, cut into ½-inch pieces

1 juicy tomato, cut into ½-inch chunks

1 red or yellow bell pepper, cut into ½-inch pieces

1-½ cups cooked corn kernels

1 cup cilantro, chopped

Place shrimp in a medium-size bowl. Add enough citrus juice so that they are entirely covered. Cover the bowl with plastic wrap and marinate the shrimp in the refrigerator for at least 30 minutes (they should appear mostly pink). When you're done marinating mix all the ingredients (including the citrus marinade, but not the cilantro) in a large bowl. Right before serving, add the cilantro.

Serving size: ¾ cup. Makes 6-8 servings.
Per serving: 75 calories; 0.5 grams fat

TIPS:

- Try other shellfish and white fish (e.g., scallops and tilapia) in place of shrimp.
- Use the freshest seafood possible or buy frozen (the seafood is generally frozen when caught, so carries minimal risk of food poisoning). If you are in doubt of the seafood's freshness, boil for 1 minute before marinating.
- Vegetarians can use chickpeas or tofu instead of shellfish.
- Add a small amount of vinegar and/or orange juice for extra flavor.

TWO BURGERS

Burgers are universally loved and practical. Make a batch on a Sunday and enjoy them through the week — they taste even better after the flavors have had a chance to blend together.

VEGGIE BURGERS

2 cups cooked black or red beans or chickpeas; or one 15-ounce can of beans (reserve some cooking liquid)

½ cup rolled oats (not instant)

1-2 onions, peeled and quartered

2-3 cloves raw or roasted garlic

1 egg

1 tablespoon parsley

1 tablespoon rosemary

1 tablespoon chili powder

Salt and freshly ground black pepper

Have on hand:

Bean-cooking liquid, stock, or other liquid (wine, milk, water, or even ketchup) if necessary to moisten

Panko crumbs or more oats if necessary to add texture

Extra-virgin olive oil or neutral oil

Combine all ingredients except liquid and oil in food processor and pulse until just combined (leave the mixture a little chunky). If the mixture is dry or crumbly, add one of the liquids suggested until the mixture is moist, not wet. If the mixture seems *too* wet, add oats and/or panko. Once you're finished adjusting, let the mixture rest for a few minutes to firm up.

With wet hands, shape mixture into six to eight patties and let rest again for a few minutes. Spray a large nonstick skillet with oil and turn heat to medium. When hot, add patties. Cook undisturbed until browned (about 5 minutes), then turn carefully with spatula and cook 3 or 4 more minutes until firm and browned. Serve with mustard, ketchup, chutney or other toppings.

TIPS:

- For a milder onion flavor, roast the onion before adding it to the mix.
- Instead of chili powder, use the spice mix of your choice.
- Both the burger mixture and shaped burgers can be covered tightly and refrigerated for up to a day. Bring back to room temperature before cooking.
- Add more veggies to reduce the calorie count. Roasted or baked veggies work best, but raw shredded carrots and chopped tomatoes also work well.

Makes 6-8 burgers. Per burger: 100-120 calories (depending on size), 1-2 grams fat
(Calorie/fat count does not include bun, toppings, and condiments)

TURKEY BURGERS

Apple gives these burgers a slightly sweet taste, and the vegetables increase the volume while decreasing the calories.

¾ pound extra-lean ground turkey

½ cup sweet apple, finely chopped

2 ripe tomatoes, chopped

1 medium-to-large yellow onion, finely chopped

1-2 carrots, shredded

¼ cup panko or bread crumbs

1 tablespoon rosemary

Salt and pepper to taste

In a large bowl combine all ingredients by hand and form into four patties. Spray the bottom of a large nonstick skillet with oil and turn heat to medium. When hot, add patties. Cook undisturbed until browned, about 5 minutes; turn carefully with spatula and cook 3 or 4 minutes until firm and browned.

> TIP: *Experiment with the amount and type of vegetables you use. I like carrots and tomatoes best, but others have enjoyed parsnips, garlic, and green onions.*

Makes 4 burgers
Per serving: 115 calories; 1 gram fat

Can I eat pizza when I'm trying to lose weight?

Pizza is high-calorie for five reasons:
1. The pizza dough is coated with oil
2. It's usually topped with lots of cheese
3. The crust is usually thick
4. The tomato sauce contains oil and sugar
5. The toppings (sausage, pepperoni, etc.) are often high in fat

HEALTHY & EASY PIZZA

You can make pizza at home that trims some of the excess and still tastes great. (See the recipe notes for the starred items in the ingredients.)

½ cup low-fat pizza sauce*

Olive oil spray

1 large garlic bulb

12-inch low-fat, thin pizza crust*

1 zucchini

1 cup green onion, chopped

1 cup mushrooms

1 tomato, sliced thin

½ cup cauliflower, sliced

1 cup fat-free shredded cheese*

Spices: basil, parsley, onion or garlic powder, salt

Preheat oven to 450°F.

Make the sauce: Remove the top from the garlic bulb so that the tips of the cloves are visible. Spritz the bulb with olive oil, then wrap it in aluminum foil and roast until soft, approximately 30 minutes. Remove from oven. When it's cool enough to touch, squeeze out the softened garlic and mix it into the pizza sauce in a small bowl or cup.

Assemble the pizza: Pre-bake the crust for 5 minutes, then pull it out of the oven and give it a quick, very light spritz of olive oil. Spread it with the sauce-garlic mixture, and layer on the veggies. Add a few dashes of spice and salt, top with the cheese, and bake until the crust is golden brown and the veggies are soft (typically 8-10 minutes). Remove from oven and let it cool. Slice and serve.

TIPS:

- You can roast the garlic in advance. If you don't use it immediately, keep the bulb intact (instead of squeezing out the cloves), wrap it in foil, and refrigerate. It will keep for a few days without drying out.

- When choosing pizza sauce, look for one with fewer than 60 calories, and no more than one gram of fat per quarter cup.

- If you choose low-fat cheese, reduce the amount to about ¾ cup. If you choose full-fat cheese, reduce the amount to ½ cup.

- Most grocery stores sell frozen pizza dough; Trader Joe's and other chains also sell it fresh. It's a much tastier option and it only takes a few extra minutes to shape the dough into a pizza.

Serving size and number will vary based on preference.
Per slice *(based on 6 slices)*: 165 calories, 3 grams fat. Whole pizza: 990 calories, 19 grams fat

Desserts

AGAR "JELLO"

Agar is a high-fiber, calorie-free powder made from algae. It is also vegan.

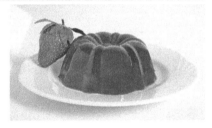

2 cups of any plain fruit juice

2 tablespoons agar flakes

Put juice in a saucepan, add agar flakes, and bring to a boil. Reduce heat to low and simmer until flakes dissolve. *Do not stir.* Pour into a mold, cupcake tins, or a baking dish (depending on your quantity) and refrigerate until set and cool.

TIPS

- Add a few slices of fruit.

- Experiment with other drinks — I've had good results with VitaminWater Zero. I also like to make this using tea sweetened with a touch of honey and stevia.

Serving size: ½ cup. Makes 6 servings.
Per serving *(average; will vary based on ingredients)*:
60 calories; 0 grams fat

HEALTHY ICE CREAM

I taught this recipe in my nutrition classes in Nicaragua. There, regular ice cream is popular but expensive, while bananas cost pennies. This recipe ends up being easy on both your health and your pocketbook.

Bananas
(1 large banana makes about 1 cup)

Optional:
Yogurt (plain or flavored)

Flavor variations:
Other frozen fruit

½ teaspoon ground cinnamon

2 tablespoons unsweetened cocoa

1 teaspoon vanilla, coconut,
or cinnamon extract

Cut bananas crosswise into ½-inch slices. Lay the slices flat on a plate or baking pan and put in the freezer. When the slices are frozen as hard as pebbles (this will take at least an hour), put them in a blender or food processor and process on high speed. In the first minute or two they will spin without breaking apart. They then might clump together and cause the machine to clog up. Pause the machine often, and manually break up the mixture when you need to. After a few minutes the mixture will turn creamy and take on a texture like ice cream. You can mix in a spoonful of plain or flavored yogurt to experiment with consistency and flavor. Add any of the suggestions from the list to flavor.

Serving size: 1 cup. Number of servings will vary.
Per serving: 100-150 calories, 0.5 grams fat
(will vary depending on what flavor additives you use)

Cooking Protein Staples: Beans, Eggs, Chicken

BEANS

While you can always use canned beans, cooking beans from scratch is fairly effortless. From-scratch beans also taste better and are much less expensive.

Soaking

Most cooks recommend soaking as it reduces cooking time and is widely believed to improve digestibility. Some people don't soak, however, claiming that unsoaked beans have better flavor. In Latin America no one soaks. This might be due to the fact that people have access to much fresher beans than we do in North America. I recommend soaking. There are two methods:

- *Overnight soak:* Rinse your beans and do a quick sort. (Occasionally a pebble or piece of dirt finds its way into a bag of beans.) Put beans in a pot with enough water to cover the beans with a few inches to spare.
- *Quick soak:* Follow the same directions as the overnight soak, then bring beans to a boil for two minutes. Let sit for at least two hours.

Cooking

1. Drain the soaking liquid and cook the beans with fresh water. A 3:1 ratio (water to beans) works well. If you have hard water, use bottled water to cook beans.

2. Add some vegetables to beans while they cook to add flavor and nutrition. Try a mixture of diced carrots, peppers (or celery), and onions.

3. In the last five minutes or so of the cooking process, when the beans are becoming soft (20-60 minutes depending on the kind of bean), add salt, tomatoes (canned or chopped fresh), herbs, and spices.

POACHED EGGS

I always poach my eggs. It's very easy, and it's the lowest-calorie method — there's no need to add fat, as you do with scrambled or fried eggs.

How-to:

1. Fill a pan with about an inch of water and bring to a simmer.

2. Crack open and add egg(s) directly to the water

3. Simmer: Four minutes will produce an egg with a firm white and a bit of a runny yolk. Five minutes will solidify the yolk.

4. Remove from the water using a slotted spoon.

BAKED CHICKEN

Baking chicken is easy and fast. Most medium-size pieces (three to four ounces) will be fully cooked in 30 minutes or less. Try roasting vegetables with the chicken for a one-pan meal.

Seasoning

Try herbs and spices like onion powder, basil, rosemary, garlic, mustard powder, thyme, paprika, cayenne pepper, and celery seed.

Marinating

The options for marinades are endless. Try using low-calorie salad dressings, and see the recipes below. Put the chicken in a resealable food storage container or plastic bag. Add two tablespoons of marinade for every four-ounce piece of chicken. Refrigerate for an hour or two. Occasionally shake or invert the container so that the marinade soaks into all parts of the chicken. When you're done, remove the chicken from the marinade and follow the instructions that follow. Discard marinade — do not use during roasting.

Cooking:

1. Preheat the oven to 425°F. Pat the chicken dry using paper towels and season, or remove from marinade. Arrange the pieces on a baking sheet or in a glass baking dish. The pieces should be skin-up, in a single layer, with space between each piece.

2. Bake for 20 to 30 minutes. The chicken is done when opaque all the way through. (You shouldn't see any pink.) You can use a cooking thermometer to check—the chicken is cooked when the thermometer registers at least 165°F in the thickest part.

3. If you'd like the skin to be crispy, turn on the broiler for 2 to 3 minutes. Watch closely to prevent overbrowning.

Marinades

I've always liked using marinades, but the first time I started using them on a daily basis was when I started working for Shane Diet & Fitness Centers in 2015. I had the challenge of providing reasonably large meals that were filling, tasted good, and were also low in calories. I found that using low-calorie marinades was the single most important factor in making the meals tasty.

ASIAN

2 tablespoons light soy sauce

2 tablespoons seasoned
rice wine vinegar

2 tablespoons minced fresh ginger

½ tablespoon sesame oil

BALSAMIC

⅓ cup balsamic vinegar

1 garlic clove, minced

2 tablespoons fresh lemon juice

1 tablespoon fresh basil, minced

1 tablespoon shallot or onion, minced

Salt and pepper to taste

CITRUS

¾ cup fresh orange juice

2 tablespoons chopped fresh basil

2 tablespoons lime juice

2 tablespoons extra-virgin olive oil

1 garlic clove, crushed

½ teaspoon dried crushed red pepper

¼ teaspoon salt

LEMON GARLIC

½ teaspoon olive oil

4 tablespoons lemon juice

1 tablespoon lemon zest

2 teaspoons minced garlic

Salt and pepper to taste

SOUTHWESTERN

1 tablespoon balsamic vinegar

2 teaspoons garlic powder

½ teaspoon oregano

1 teaspoon paprika

½ teaspoon cumin

Mix the ingredients together and add your choice of protein or vegetables. See the marinating instructions for Baked Chicken (previous page) for more tips. Marinate for at least an hour before cooking. Discard the marinade when you're ready to cook—do not reuse it or cook with it.

Sprouting

The seeds of a variety of plant foods can be sprouted — nuts, seeds, grains, beans, and vegetables. If you're new to sprouting, I recommend that you begin with the easiest seeds to sprout: radish, pea, chickpea, mung bean, alfalfa, fenugreek, sunflower, lentil, and broccoli. These are available at most health food stores and from a variety of online retailers.

There are five steps to sprouting:

1. Place seeds in a container and add warm water, cover with a cloth, and let soak at room temperature overnight. The water-to-seed ratio should be about 2:1. Rinse thoroughly and drain.

2. Prepare a quart-size or larger Mason jar (or any wide-mouth canning jar). To allow for easier draining, remove the solid-metal insert from the lid. When you're ready to seal the jar, drape a piece of cheesecloth (or any kind of breathable cloth) over the top of the jar, and screw the lid on over the cloth. Alternatively, you can drill a few little holes in the metal lid.

3. Fill one-third of the jar with your presoaked seeds, and fill the rest of the jar with warm or room-temperature water. Put the lid or fabric on the jar, then drain the water. Your seeds should be damp, but not swimming in water.

4. Rinse and repeat: To keep your seeds at the right moisture level and inhibit mold growth, you'll need to rinse the seeds two to three times a day. Follow the same basic procedure as in the previous step: Remove the lid, fill the jar with room-temperature or warm water, replace the lid, and drain the water. Do this until the sprouts are ready: for most sprouts this is when you see sprouts of an inch or more — usually in two to five days.

5. Enjoy! Sprouts can be a low-calorie addition to tacos, salads, sandwiches, and wraps. They're also tasty as a fresh topping to soups and stews or on their own, (lightly) steamed.

Health caveat: As with other raw and unpasteurized foods — oysters, sushi, eggs, milk, cheese — sprouts are occasionally found to be a source of unhealthy bacteria (like varieties of *E. coli* and Salmonella), and can cause food poisoning. The risk of purchasing contaminated seeds is minimal, but if you have a compromised immune system it is best to check with your physician before making sprouts a regular part of your diet.

Acknowledgments

Writing a book is a collaborative process and I was fortunate to have a great deal of assistance. The core team of professional collaborators who spent countless hours helping me are acknowledged later in this section; here I would like to thank all the others who made this book possible. So many of them—for instance, the countless kind and generous Nicaraguans whom I worked with, taught, interviewed, and befriended—can't be named. Among those I can readily name and thank are the following friends, family, and institutions:

A core group of family served as kitchen-table editors, cheerleaders, and motivators: my parents, Charles and Lizou Fenyvesi; my brother and sister-in-law, Shamu Fenyvesi Sadeh and Jaime Sadeh (my relentless, stellar editors, especially early on); my sister, Malka Fenyvesi; and my brother-in-law, Alex Kroll.

Jimmy Grisham helped me with early ideas about basic layout and design. Lisa Davidowitz and Jennifer Matoney did a wonderful job editing my manuscript in its rough-draft stage.

I'd like to thank several good friends, without whose support I would never been able to finish this book: Mark Lorenz and Richard Palmer-Smith, both of whom visited me in Nicaragua; Mary Cobb, who connected me with my illustrator; and Eithne McMenamin and Emma Hambright, who gave me many good ideas.

Three authors gave me insightful feedback on writing and publishing: Liz Lipiski, Ed Ugel, and Erica Jong. Mrs. Jong was particularly instrumental in editing the first two chapters and suggesting that I start the book with my personal journey.

Other friends and colleagues who helped along the way: My friend and former bandmate, Todd McCloskey, gave me ideas for quotes for starting chapters. Former Peace Corps volunteers Curt Davis and Lara Gunderson were my housemates in Managua while they were working on their Nicaragua-related PhDs. They were full of insightful critiques that helped me as I wrote. Jovannia Chamorro Padilla and Dona Marta were my neighbors in Managua and they did a wonderful job hosting the volunteers for my Fulbright program. Patricia Rodriguez, a former Nicaraguan revolutionary, was my housemate in San Francisco, and offered valuable cultural insights.

Many thanks to the Pellas family and Los Rayos Restaurant, where I often ate and where I always enjoyed the company; we filmed much of the documentary short that accompanies this book at the restaurant.

A very special thank you to the U.S. State Department and the Fulbright Program, whose staff includes Maira Vargas, Jennifer Fox, and Steve Huneke. Also, to all the incredibly welcoming and easy-to-work-with staff at The National Autonomous University of Nicaragua (UNAN) in Managua: Kenia Paramo; Juan Francisco Rocha, Director del Instituto Politécnico de la Salud; Ana María Gutiérrez Carcache, Directora del Departamento de Nutrición; Lucrecia del Rosario Arias, Jenny del Carmen Casco Palma, Violeta Carvajal Marenco, Vilma Rosa Perez, Ligia Pasquier Guerrero, Carmen Maria Flores Machado, and Linda Solórzano Benedit. And a heartfelt thank you to all my students at UNAN, especially "los monos" at La Vida en Equilbrio: Ariel Cristiana Marín, Taimy Hernández, Diego Gabriel Castro Navarro, Lillie Orozco, Carlos Aburto Gonzalez, and Bell Gadea. James Womack and Vida en Equilibrio in Popoyo also hosted a pivotal workshop retreat for my project.

To my colleagues in the international aid community:

Dawson Farr and Tabitha Parker from Natural Doctors International, where I volunteered many times, were key sounding boards for my ideas on Nicaragua's nutrition transition. Peace Corps Nicaragua invited me to conduct a few trainings, where I learned as much as I taught. The Peace Corps also helped me make invaluable local contacts. Vision Inclusiva, a Nicaraguan nonprofit that works on chronic disease, was a fascinating place to volunteer. I learned a great deal there. Susan Kinne and Grupo Fenix, who hosted my first volunteer experience in 2002 and whom I remained in close communication with over the years. Thanks to Tim Gibb and Global Community Innovations, who worked together with Namlo on the study I describe in Chapter 15. Thanks to everyone who volunteered under my

Fulbright grant, kept my spirits up, and were full of great energy and ideas: Hilary McHone, Eliza Jane Oatz, Fausto Ruiz, Janelle Ruiz, Deji Jaiyesimi, Sarah Canal, Shanon Sidell, Dana Martell, Emily Brumstead, Tanya Havin, and Ronja Geyser.

To my colleagues in the health and wellness community:

La Clinica de La Raza, in Oakland, California, greatly accelerated my interest in and knowledge of Latino health issues. I am grateful to all of their staff and, in particular, my dietitian mentor Joan Thompson. I am grateful to Project Open Hand in Oakland where I learned about more about the nutrition needs of HIV and cancer patients and to DaVita Dialysis in Washington, D.C., where the mix of patients has presented me with many opportunities for growth and learning.

Rancho La Puerta, where I worked off and on for several years was instrumental in my progress as a writer and dietitian. I attended many fascinating lectures there and was lucky to have collaborated on lectures and menus with their staff nutritionist Yvonne Nienstadt and program manager Barry Shingle. Shane Diet and Weight Loss Resorts, where I have worked for the past three summers was a great place to test out many of my menu and lecture ideas, and I learned so much working with hundreds of the programs' attendees. I am grateful to owners David Ettenberg and Ziporah Janowski.

Wellspring Weight Loss Camps, where I spent four summers, was another formative learning experience and I am grateful for the program's directors: Lynne Papa, Eliza Kingsford, and Jude Wood.

I also want to thank my favorite yoga instructor, Katie Papo, who I had the pleasure of working with at both Wellspring and Shane.

To my colleagues in academics:

Bastyr University gave me my first grant to go to Nicaragua. I learned so much at Bastyr, and I am thankful for the support and inspiration from their professors and my fellow students. Thanks to Doris Picinin, Kelly Morrow, Erica M., Kelly Hanna, and Katherine McCauley.

Marsha Piacun, the dietetic internship director at Tulane University always encouraged my interest in Latino health issues and ran a superb internship program. Another mentor that both encouraged and influenced me greatly was Sara Ducy, a longtime nutrition professor and resource to so many students at Montgomery College.

To my musician friends:

I'm a barely proficient musician, no more, but I've had the pleasure of playing with so many brilliant musicians whose talent and friendship has meant the world to me. There are far too many to name but, at the least, one grand shout out goes to my most consistent fellowship-of-the-stringsters: John and Jill Turpin, Jason and Erin Frigerio, Tim Ryan and Daniella Fischetti.

And finally:

For two years now I have struggled to describe the entire extent of Anastasia Miller's role. I would describe her to friends and family as the best editor, graphic designer, illustrator, and photographer, and when I ran out of words I would say she is the "guru of all things book related." I hired her in 2015 when I was looking for a designer for Chapter 3 and the Appendix—at a time when I was sure the book was almost done. While she was reading the first few chapters she flagged some typos and copyediting issues and asked if I wanted her to review the rest of the book. I braced myself and agreed. She came back with pages of notes; first accompanying her suggestions with a "you don't *have* to do this" disclaimer, and then digging deeper and noting places in which I could improve the flow with a different approach or technique, or sometimes just start from scratch. As we discussed content and flow she encouraged me to incorporate more material from my time in Nicaragua. She gave the same attention to all the visual elements of the book. While she kept elements of the design I'd developed with my first creative team, she reviewed every illustration, photograph, and graphic for clarity and effectiveness. Whether she was suggesting a caption or section title, photographing tablespoons of hummus and piles of pepper flakes, or creating dozens of options for the layout of various complex pages, she was game for whatever it took to make the book as good as it could possibly be. She always treated this book with the same care as if it were her own; she is a true collaborator.

Photo and Illustration Credits

One of the things that makes this book stand out is the contribution of the talented artists and photographers whose work brightens these pages. I extend my sincere thanks to everyone who allowed their work to be published here.

Photography

PHOTOGRAPHER	PAGE(S)
Michelle Blondin Blanz	10 (left)
Darrell Bushnell	156
Curt Davis	24 (top)
Alexandra D'Elia	33 (bottom)
Jessica Dell'Aquila	36 (bottom)
Tim Gibb	23 (middle), (bottom left), 181 (top right), 182, 187
Mathew Karsten	105
Renee Kelemen	viii
Susan Kinne	23 (bottom), 44 (bottom)
Fritz Liedtke	143
Mark Lorenz	6, 14
Ariel Cristiana Marín	181 (left)
Lisa McKinney	40 (middle)
Anastasia Miller	ii, ix, 97, 98
Jenny Moran	vi (left), 32 (middle, bottom), 33 (middle), 34 (middle, bottom), 35 (middle, bottom), 37 (top, bottom), 38 (top, middle), 42, 144
Pam Moran	v
Dana Mortell	96 (top), 99, 127 (bottom)
Liza Jane Oatz	41 (right), 132, 159
Jovannia Chamorro Padilla	vi (right)
Kenia Paramo	170
Jay Ruzicka	37 (middle)
Annie Schwarcz	xi
Lindsay Schwartz	39
Shutterstock	Julija Dmitrijeva, cover; Simon Dannhauer, 8; Michel Sabbagh, 202; Syda Productions, 110; Nikkytok, 137; Africa Studio, 152 (pepper grinder); Simply Photos, 123; Everett Historical, 122 (bottom); Zkruger, 122 (top left); withgod, 122 (top right); Brooke Becker, 40 (bottom right); stockcreations, 40 (bottom left); Olga Nayashkova, 40 (top plate); Jacek Chabraszewsk, 40 (bottom plate)
Sarah Twitchell	7, back cover
Denise Van Wissen	19 (bottom)
Natalie Irene Woodrum	16, 66, 166

My own photographs appear on pages 1, 10 (right), 11, 19 (top), 23 (top) 24 (bottom right), 32 (top), 33 (top), 34 (top), 35 (top), 36 (middle), 38 (bottom), 41 (left), 44 (top), 53 (bottom), 68, 69, 79, 84, 89, 92, 96 (bottom), 108, 114, 127 (top), 173, 181 (bottom right)

Illustrations and Graphics

The illustrations Jenny Moran and I worked on together evolved as the book did. Jenny created original illustrations except where noted; Anastasia Miller art-directed or reworked Jenny's illustrations where noted.

Original concepts/direction: Dan Fenyvesi; Illustrations: Jenny Moran

Reworked Illustrations

Original concepts: Dan Fenyvesi; Illustrations: Jenny Moran
Rework: Anastasia Miller

Reworked Illustrations (cont'd)

Graphics and Illustration by Anastasia Miller

Original concepts: Dan Fenyvesi, except where marked

The Food Sobriety Team

Design and Editorial

MICHAL KEELEY *(copy editing)* is a mostly retired editor and journalist who has happily forsaken city life for the country. During a 35-year career in the D.C. area, she worked for both government agencies and news organizations such as the *Washington Post, U.S. News & World Report, Salon,* and *Politico.* She was fortunate enough to meet the multi-talented Anastasia Miller when they were both employed by the Peace Corps, and she is delighted to have had the chance to work with her again. While working on this book, Michal was inspired to eat a healthier diet and looks forward to trying some of the recipes.

ANASTASIA MILLER *(book layout and production, illustration, photography, art cleanup, developmental editing and writing, recipe testing and troubleshooting)* is a Washington, D.C.-based freelance creative director, designer, and copy editor. For the last 15 years she has used her communications skills in aid of international volunteerism and relief; public health, homelessness, and U.S. healthcare; and many other public policy issues.

For Anastasia this project began as a quick layout gig, but morphed into a 28-month coaching, editing, writing, and design journey to help Dan realize his vision for the book. In support of that effort she spent a year (and count-ing) re-learning Spanish, adopted the Food Sobriety philosophy, and com-pletely changed the way she cooks and eats. She can enthusiastically vouch for the Sober Plate method—she lost 25 pounds in the endeavor and has kept that extra weight off for more than one year.

JENNY RODRIGUEZ MORAN *(illustration, photography)* is a portrait artist, illustrator and photographer. She loves to paint pictures and plates with lines, words, fresh ingredients and color. Join Jenny's adventures and browse her storied pages as an artist, culinary dabbler and new momma on her site: www.StudioJenMoran.com

Edición en Español

YOLANDA PAREDES *(translation)* is a naturopathic doctor with a focus on helping people get healthy with food and lifestyle changes. She has a B.S. in chemistry from UC Berkeley and received her naturopathic degree from Bastyr University. She has worked in Mexico in private practice and as a nutrition specialist developing school lunch programs and training staff in nutrition education and food preparation. She enjoys working directly with communities to promote food awareness and the importance of a healthy diet. Taking her kids on walks and runs is one of the highlights of her day.

ELIZABETH TREVIÑO *(translation)* from Monterrey, Mexico holds a bachelor's degree in Spanish literature and is in her last year as a Ph.D. candidate in Spanish philology at the Autonomous University of Barcelona, Spain. For more than a decade, in addition to her academic work, she has dedicated herself to editorial pursuits and publishing, working with publishing companies including Random House Mondadori.

Documentary Film Short

KEVIN NAPIER is a writer, filmmaker, and improviser. Kevin produced the documentary short that accompanies this book, "A Faustian Bargain." His work has been shown at South by Southwest, the Aspen Comedy Arts Fest, the New York Television Festival, and the Santa Fe, Santa Barbara, and Palm Springs film festivals. As a writer he has worked with Gary Sanchez (Will Ferrell and Adam McKay's company), Red Hour (Ben Stiller's production company), among others, and has sold shows to ABC, NBC, FX, and Fox, including creating and co-executive producing the Fox TV pilot "The Station." He wrote for the recent FX series "Married" and has two series in development with Showtime and Amazon. He has also studied and performed improv for the past 10 years and developed improv to scripted videos in New York City, Bangalore, Barcelona, and Berlin.

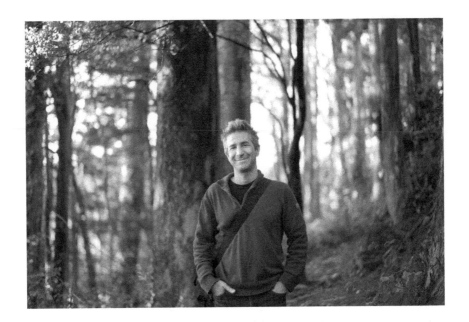

About the Author

Dan Fenyvesi teaches nutrition at Montgomery College in Rockville, Maryland and works as a renal dietitian for DaVita in Washington, D.C. In addition to his time in the health field, Fenyvesi's eclectic life has included installing solar panels in California (with the Solar Living Institute in Hopland and Occidental Power in San Francisco) and in Spain (as a "WOOFER," with Willing Workers on Organic Farms); teaching English in Budapest, and touring the U.S. playing bass in the jam bands The Floodplain Gang and The McCloskey Brothers Band. While working in Nicaragua, Fenyvesi occasionally filled in on guitar for the reggae bands James Sedgwick and Los Pobrecitos (in San Juan Del Sur), and Philip Montalbán (in Managua).

Fenyvesi also enjoys volunteering. In the U.S. he has participated with the Democratic party and HeadCount in get-out-the-vote efforts. He has collaborated with international nonprofit and governmental groups whose missions he wholeheartedly supports, including Grupo Fenix, Natural Doctors International, Namlo, the Peace Corps, and Vision Inclusiva. Fenyvesi hopes to use *Food Sobriety* and his documentary short "A Faustian Bargain" as platforms to spark dialogue, increase awareness, and work toward improved health and social justice in Latin America and the United States.